Essential
Examination

2nd Edition Essential Examination

Step-by-step system-based guide to clinical examination
with practical tips and key facts for OSCEs

Alasdair K B Ruthven MBChB (Hons) BSc (Hons)

Foundation Year 2 Doctor

Royal Infirmary, Edinburgh, UK

Scion

© Scion Publishing Ltd, 2010

ISBN 978 1 904842 84 2

First published in 2010

A CIP catalogue record for this book is available from the British Library.

Scion Publishing Limited
The Old Hayloft, Vantage Business Park, Bloxham Road, Banbury, Oxfordshire OX16 9UX
www.scionpublishing.com

Important Note from the Publisher
The information contained within this book was obtained by Scion Publishing Limited from sources believed by us to be reliable. However, while every effort has been made to ensure its accuracy, no responsibility for loss or injury whatsoever occasioned to any person acting or refraining from action as a result of information contained herein can be accepted by the author or publishers.

Readers should remember that medicine is a constantly evolving science and while the author and publishers have ensured that all dosages, applications and practices are based on current indications, there may be specific practices which differ between communities. You should always follow the guidelines laid down by the manufacturers of specific products and the relevant authorities in the country in which you are practising.

Although every effort has been made to ensure that all owners of copyright material have been acknowledged in this publication, we would be pleased to acknowledge in subsequent reprints or editions any omissions brought to our attention.

Typeset by Phoenix Photosetting, Chatham, Kent, UK
Printed by The Complete Product Company, Malmesbury, UK

CONTENTS

PREFACE

BACKGROUND

Essential Examination began life as a set of notes I produced for my undergraduate exams. At that time I was unable to find an examination skills book that succinctly laid out the full sequence for examination of one body system on one page. This format remains the basis of this new edition, which has steadily expanded over the past 5 years. Although the content has been extensively reviewed, refined and updated, much of the information is still presented in ways which helped me to remember it at medical school.

GENERIC FORMAT

Each system-based examination described has its own double-page spread (with the exception of cranial nerves, which needed two). The first spread comprises a clear, step-by-step guide to examining that particular patient, including useful things to say to the patient (or an examiner), detailed descriptions of special tests, etc. Contained in the right-hand column is a collection of key information: potential findings, differential diagnoses of clinical signs and practical tips. On the following spread is a series of facts relating to that particular examination, selected because of the regularity with which they are asked about in bedside teaching and OSCEs. In some sections there are also tips on how to present your findings succinctly – we all know how easy it is to lose our way here.

WHAT'S NOT INCLUDED

To use this book requires a good baseline understanding of the physiology and pathophysiology of the systems considered. Some detail has been omitted intentionally – for example, nowhere is the exact method of examining for flapping tremor explained. It is assumed that core skills like this become second nature as they are taught time and time again in clinical teaching. This makes space for other useful information, and detailed descriptions of less familiar elements of examination where the margins between looking slick and looking awkward are smaller. Often there are many ways of examining for the same thing in medicine; in such cases I have described either the method preferred by specialists, or where no consensus exists, the method which I find the easiest.

HOW TO USE THIS BOOK

To get the most out of *Essential Examination* first familiarise yourself with the examinations and learn some of the associated facts. Then the key is *practice*. Spend as much time as you can with fellow students examining patients (and each other), and quizzing one another on the information in the right-hand columns and on the notes for each section. Remember that usually you should examine from the patient's right-hand side, although some examinations (especially orthopaedic) require you to move around the bed.

A NOTE ON EXAMS

More often than not in clinical exams you will not be asked to complete the full examination of a particular body system. Instead, you may be asked to complete part of that examination (rather than 'examine the cardiovascular system', simply 'examine the precordium', for example). However, in order to do this you must draw from a baseline knowledge of the examination in its entirety. Alternatively you may be asked to examine multiple systems at once (e.g. a cardio-respiratory examination). *Always* listen to what the examiner asks. It is also important to remember that many examinations follow a similar sequence, in particular:

- Core medical: peripheral signs → inspection → palpation → percussion → auscultation
- Neurology: inspection → tone → power → reflexes → sensation → co-ordination
- Orthopaedics: look → feel → move → special tests → check distal neurovascular integrity

If you get lost in an examination (which is easy to do under the pressure of assessment), default to these basic frameworks to get yourself back on track. Some examinations, of course, follow their own unique sequence; these are the most difficult to learn and so you should become very familiar with them. Always have some concluding remarks up your sleeve too – it's a good way to finish off, and gives the impression that you really know your stuff.

Finally, remember that in order to pass you do not need to recall every single piece of information contained in this book – a slick, comprehensive clinical examination combined with some solid core knowledge is certainly enough. The old saying that difficult questions mean you are doing well is very true – don't forget it!

If you have any questions or comments regarding the book, please email me at: author@essentialexamination.com

Best of luck in all of your studies.

A.K.B. Ruthven
July 2010

ACKNOWLEDGEMENTS

I would like to thank my many clinical tutors and senior colleagues for their role in the creation and development of this book. In particular, Mr Mark Gaston for his help with the orthopaedic sections, Mr Zahid Raza for reviewing the vascular sections, Dr Ingibjorg Gudmundsdottir for her input into the cardiology sections, and Dr Kirsty Dundas for her help with the pregnant abdomen section.

I would also like to express my appreciation for all the undergraduates who have supported the project with their recommendations and abundant enthusiasm.

FOREWORD

The most important core skills for medical students to master are history taking and clinical examination. This conveniently pocket-sized, ring-bound text has been written with the philosophy that clinical skills can be more effectively honed at the bedside, and as such it should be used as a constant companion on the ward and in the consulting room.

Each section of the book covers the physical examination of a body system, beginning with a detailed step-by-step description of the examination method, complemented by practical tips and key facts. Detailed information relating to that examination is provided in the form of helpful illustrations, diagrams and tables with space for you to add your own notes.

This book is intended primarily to be used by medical students in their 'clinical' years who, having attained a sound grasp of clinical science and disease processes are beginning to hone examination techniques. It is of particular use to those who are preparing for final assessments and practising techniques during revision.

Professor Mike Ford
Edinburgh, 2010

ABBREVIATIONS

Shorthand

ΔΔ	Differential diagnosis	2°	Secondary to
#	Fracture	Ca	Cancer
♂	Male	Pt	Patient
♀	Female	Rx	Treatment
[pxx]	See page xx	[↻]	See over: check in Notes

Alphabetical list of abbreviations

AAA	Abdominal aortic aneurysm	LMN	Lower motor neurone
ABG	Arterial blood gas	LLSE	Lower left sternal edge
ABPI	Ankle brachial pressure index	LSV	Long saphenous vein
AC	Acromio-clavicular (joint)	LV	Left ventricle
ACEi	ACE inhibitor	LVH	Left ventricular hypertrophy
ACL	Anterior cruciate ligament (of knee)	MCL	Medial collateral ligament (of knee)
ACTH	Adrenocorticotrophic hormone	MI	Myocardial infarction
AF	Atrial fibrillation	MND	Motor neurone disease
A–P	Anterior–posterior (diameter)	MNG	Multinodular goitre
APKD	Adult polycystic kidney disease	MR	Mitral regurgitation
AR	Aortic regurgitation	MRA	Magnetic resonance angiography
AS	Aortic stenosis	MRI	Magnetic resonance imaging (scan)
ASIS	Anterior superior iliac spine	MS	Mitral stenosis / Multiple sclerosis
AV	Arterio-venous (malformation / fistula)	NOF	Neck of femur (fracture)
AVN	Avascular necrosis	NSAID	Non-steroidal anti-inflammatory drug
BP	Blood pressure	OA	Osteoarthritis
CABG	Coronary artery bypass graft	OCP	Oral contraceptive pill
CCF	Congestive cardiac failure	PBC	Primary biliary cirrhosis
CDH	Congenital dislocation of the hip	PCA	Posterior communicating artery
CFA	Cryptogenic fibrosing alveolitis	PCL	Posterior cruciate ligament (of knee)
CHD	Congenital heart disease	PE	Pulmonary embolism
CKD	Chronic kidney disease	PFTs	Pulmonary function tests
CLD	Chronic liver disease	PIPJ	Proximal interphalangeal joint
CML	Chronic myeloid leukaemia	PND	Paroxysmal nocturnal dyspnoea
CN	Cranial nerve	PNS	Peripheral nervous system
CNS	Central nervous system	PR	Pulmonary regurgitation / Per-rectal (examination)
COPD	Chronic obstructive pulmonary disease	PSC	Primary sclerosing cholangitis
CRP	C-reactive protein	PVD	Peripheral vascular disease

CRF	Chronic renal failure	R-R	Radio-radial (delay)
CRT	Capillary refill time	RA	Rheumatoid arthritis
CSF	Cerebrospinal fluid	RAAS	Renin–angiotensin–aldosterone system
CT	Computerised tomography (scan)	RAPD	Relative afferent papillary defect
CXR	Chest X-ray	RHF	Right heart failure
DHS	Dynamic hip screw	RIF	Right iliac fossa
DIPJ	Distal interphalangeal joint	ROM	Range of motion
DM	Diabetes mellitus	RTA	Road traffic accident
DMARD	Disease-modifying anti-rheumatic drug	RUQ	Right upper quadrant
DMD	Duchenne muscular dystrophy	RVH	Right ventricular hypertrophy
DVT	Deep vein thrombosis	SBP	Spontaneous bacterial peritonitis
EAA	Extrinsic allergic alveolitis	SC	Subcutaneous
EBV	Epstein–Barr virus	SCDC	Subacute combined degeneration of the cord
ECG	Electrocardiogram	SCLC	Small-cell lung cancer
ESR	Erythrocyte sedimentation rate	SCM	Sternocleidomastoid
FAP	Familial adenomatous polyposis	SE	Side-effects
FNA	Fine needle aspiration	SLE	Systemic lupus erythematosus
GCA	Giant cell arteritis	SOB	Shortness of breath
GFR	Glomerular filtration rate	SFJ	Sapheno-femoral junction
GH	Growth hormone	SPJ	Sapheno-popliteal junction
GI	Gastrointestinal	SaO_2	Arterial oxygen saturation
GTN	Gliceryl trinitrate (spray)	SSV	Short saphenous vein
HB	Heart block	SUFE	Slipped upper femoral epiphysis
HCC	Hepatocellular carcinoma	SVC	Superior vena cava
HOCM	Hypertrophic obstructive cardiomyopathy	TAH	Total abdominal hysterectomy
HS	Heart sound	TB	Tuberculosis
HTN	Hypertension	TFTs	Thyroid function tests
IBD	Inflammatory bowel disease	TIPSS	Transjugular intrahepatic porto-systemic shunt
ICD	Implantable cardioverter-defibrillator	TR	Tricuspid regurgitation
IE	Infective endocarditis	TS	Tricuspid stenosis
ILD	Interstitial lung disease	TSH	Thyroid stimulating hormone
IM	Intramuscular	U+Es	Urea and electrolytes
INO	Intranuclear ophthalmoplegia	UC	Ulcerative colitis
IVDU	Intravenous drug user	UMN	Upper motor neurone
JVP	Jugular venous pulse	USS	Ultrasound scan
LCL	Lateral collateral ligament (of knee)	VEB	Ventricular ectopic beat
LHF	Left heart failure	VR	Vocal resonance
LHS	Left-hand side	VSD	Ventricular septal defect
LIF	Left iliac fossa	VT	Ventricular tachycardia
LIMA	Left internal mammary artery	WCC	White cell count

MEDICINE

1. CARDIOVASCULAR SYSTEM

Action / Examine for	ΔΔ / Potential findings / Extra information
Introduction	
• Wash hands • Introduce yourself, explain examination & gain consent • Expose & position pt (top off, supine at 45°)	→ Bra should be removed for complete examination of ♀
End of bed	
• Appearance – unwell / distressed / in pain • Oxygen, fluids & medications	→ GTN spray especially
Hands	
• Feel temperature & check capillary refill time • Peripheral cyanosis • Tendon xanthomata • Osler's nodes & Janeway lesions	→ Warm & well perfused or peripherally shut down (CRT>2 sec) → PVD, Raynaud's, CCF or with central cyanosis [⇨] → Hypercholesterolaemia → IE [p9 – you could also mention Roth spots here]
Nails	
• Finger clubbing (look carefully) • Koilonychia • Splinter haemorrhages • Nailfold infarcts	→ IE, cyanotic CHD, atrial myxoma, etc. [p112] → Iron deficiency anaemia → IE, trauma (e.g. gardening, joinery) → Vasculitis, SLE
Wrist	

• Radial pulse
  ○ Rate (time over 15 sec)
  ○ Rhythm
  ○ Volume
  ○ Character
• Collapsing pulse
  ○ *"Is your shoulder sore at all?"*
  ○ Grasp pt's right wrist with your right hand, place your metacarpal heads over pt's radial artery
  ○ Support pt's elbow with your left hand
  ○ Lift their arm up above their head
• Radio-radial & radio-femoral delay
	→ Tachycardia / bradycardia
	→ Regular / irregular / irregularly irregular
	→ Normal / thready / bounding
	→ Bisferiens pulse (mixed AR/AS), slow rising pulse (AS)
	→ AR
	
	→ A collapsing pulse will thrust against your palm
	→ Cervical rib (R-R), aortic dissection / coarctation, embolism

Arm	
• *"I would now measure BP"* (in both arms if R-R delay)	→ Pulse pressure (AR wide, AS narrow)
Face	
• Malar flush	→ Mitral stenosis
Eyes	
• Corneal arcus & xanthelasma • Conjunctival pallor	→ Hypercholesterolaemia → Anaemia
Mouth	
• Central cyanosis • Poor dentition	→ Lung disease, cardiac shunt, abnormal Hb [⇨] → Risk factor for IE
Neck	

• Carotid pulse
  ○ Look for exaggerated pulsation (*Corrigan's sign*)
  ○ Briefly palpate
	→ AR
	→ Useful for assessing pulse character

- JVP → [⇨]
  - Pt at 45°, head turned slightly to right, well-lit → Don't turn head too far – you want neck muscles to relax
  - Look for double pulsation on left side of neck → Easier to see on left as you look *across* pulsation
  - Estimate height above sternal angle in cm → Normally <3–4 cm
  - *"Do you have a sore stomach at all?"*
  - Push on RUQ and watch neck to see JVP rise → Hepatojugular reflux (increased venous return from liver)
  - Check JVP rapidly falls back down → Persistent elevation of JVP indicates RHF / volume overload

The Precordium

Inspection	• Scars	
	○ Pacemaker / ICD under either clavicle	→ May be an obvious underlying lump – feel if unsure
	○ Midline sternotomy	→ CABG, valve replacement
	○ Left submammary (lift breast to check in ♀)	→ Mitral valvotomy, pericardial window
	○ Legs (if midline sternotomy look now!)	→ Vein harvesting – gives clues to previous surgery [⇨]
	• Visible heave	→ Apical (LVH) or parasternal (RVH)
Palpation	• Apex beat	→ Normally in the 5th intercostal space, midclavicular line
	○ Locate & physically count rib spaces	→ If unable to locate, consider why [⇨]
	○ Assess character	→ Tapping (MS), heaving [LVH ΔΔ ⇨], thrusting (MR/AR, LVF)
	• Left parasternal heave	→ Right ventricular hypertrophy
	• Thrills	→ Palpable murmur – grade 4 or above by definition [p9]
Auscultation (*always* whilst palpating the carotid pulse) **B – Bell** **D – Diaphragm**	• 4 primary valve areas	
	○ Apex (Mitral) – **B** then **D**	
	○ LLSE (Tricuspid) – **D**	
	○ 2nd left intercostal space (Pulmonary) – **D**	
	○ 2nd right intercostal space (Aortic) – **D**	
	• Areas of murmur radiation	
	○ Axilla – **D**	→ MR
	○ Each carotid in turn, breath held in expiration – **D**	→ AS (hold your breath too so you know when pt must breathe)
	• Manoeuvres to amplify diastolic murmurs	
	○ Apex, pt on LHS, breath held in expiration – **B**	→ Amplifies MS (note also tends to amplify MR)
	○ LLSE, pt sitting forward, breath held in expiration – **D**	→ Amplifies AR (note also tends to amplify AS)

Back	• Auscultate lung bases for crepitations	→ LHF
	• Palpate for sacral oedema	→ RHF
Ankles	• Peripheral oedema	→ RHF, numerous other causes [p113]

Concluding remarks	• Review the observation chart (BP, temperature, SaO$_2$)	
	• Abdominal examination & peripheral pulses	→ Hepatomegaly & ascites (RHF), splenomegaly (IE), AAA
	• Investigations: ECG, CXR, echocardiogram, urinalysis	→ Microscopic haematuria (IE)

Cardiac surgery scars give you clues during examination
- Midline sternotomy + leg scar = simple CABG most likely, possible valve replacement with CABG
- Midline sternotomy with no leg scar = valve replacement highly likely, possible CABG without vein graft (LIMA or radial artery)

Key JVP abnormalities
- Elevated   RHF, volume overload, PE, constrictive pericarditis
- Elevated with ↓BP   Tension pneumothorax, cardiac tamponade, massive PE
- Elevated & fixed   SVC obstruction
- Cannon A waves   Complete heart block, VEBs, VT
- Giant V waves   TR (look for ear-wiggling, feel for pulsatile hepatomegaly)

Differentiating between types of cyanosis
- Pure peripheral cyanosis causes *cold* blue hands
- Central cyanosis causes blue lips and tongue, and when severe can also cause blue hands (usually *warm*)

ΔΔ Central cyanosis (blue lips & tongue)
- Hypoxic lung disease
- Right-to-left cardiac shunt
  - Cyanotic congenital heart disease
  - Eisenmenger's syndrome
- Methaemoglobinaemia
  - Drugs
  - Toxins

ΔΔ Irregularly irregular pulse
- AF
- Ventricular ectopic beats (VEBs)
- Complete HB + variable ventricular escape

To differentiate between AF and VEBs without an ECG you can exercise the pt – this will abolish VEBs but AF will remain

Six important causes of AF
- Ischaemic heart disease
- Rheumatic heart disease
- Thyrotoxicosis
- Pneumonia
- PE
- Alcohol

ΔΔ Peripheral cyanosis (blue hands)
- Peripheral vascular disease
- Raynaud's syndrome
- Heart failure
- Shock
- (Central cyanosis when severe)

Some causes of an absent radial pulse
- Congenital (usually bilateral)
- Arterial embolism (e.g. due to AF)
- Atheroma (usually subclavian)
- Previous arterial line
- Previous coronary angiography
- Cervical rib
- Coarctation of the aorta

NOTES

Pulsus paradoxus
- An exaggeration of the normal situation in which BP falls during inspiration, to such an extent that during inspiration the peripheral pulse may not be felt despite the LV contracting (and heart sounds still being heard)
- Causes: tamponade, constrictive pericarditis, restrictive cardiomyopathy, severe obstructive lung disease

Kussmaul's sign
- A rise in the JVP on inspiration, which is the opposite of normal (and due to impaired RV filling)
- Causes: tamponade, constrictive pericarditis, restrictive cardiomyopathy

Causes of a non-palpable apex beat
1. Something is between your fingers and the apex
    - Adipose tissue (obese pt)
    - Air (pneuothorax or emphysema)
    - Fluid (pleural or pericardial effusion)
2. The apex is not in its normal position
    - Displaced (usually laterally in LHF)
    - Dextrocardia

CCF = biventricular failure = LHF + RHF

ΔΔ Heaving apex (LVH)
- Aortic stenosis
- Hypertension
- HOCM
- Coarctation of the aorta

CXR features of LHF (ABCDE)
- **A**lveolar oedema
- Kerley **B** lines
- **C**ardiomegaly
- Upper lobe venous **D**iversion
- Pleural **E**ffusion

Causes of pericarditis
- Viral (Coxsackie)
- Bacterial / fungal infection
- Immediately post-MI
- Dressler's syndrome (2–10 weeks post-MI)
- SLE / RA / scleroderma
- Uraemia
- Malignancy

3rd heart sound
- Due to rapid ventricular filling
- May be normal if <30 years old
- Think *volume overload*
- Causes: CCF, MR, AR, large anterior MI

4th heart sound
- Due to poorly compliant ventricle
- Always abnormal
- Cannot occur in AF (requires atrial contraction)
- Think *pressure overload*
- Causes: AS, HTN, HOCM, post-MI fibrosis

Causes of cardiac failure
1. Pump failure
    - IHD
    - Cardiomyopathy
    - Constrictive pericarditis
    - Arrhythmia
    - Iatrogenic (negative inotropes)
2. Excessive preload
    - Regurgitant valvular disease (MR / AR)
    - Fluid overload (renal failure, IV fluids)
3. Excessive afterload
    - AS
    - HTN
4. Isolated RHF
    - Cor pulmonale
    - Primary pulmonary HTN
5. High-output failure (rare)
    - Anaemia
    - Pregnancy
    - Metabolic (hyperthyroidism, Paget's)

NOTES

	Mitral stenosis	Mitral regurgitation
Aetiology	• Rheumatic heart disease (99%)	• Rheumatic heart disease • IE • Valve prolapse • Papillary muscle rupture (e.g. MI) • LV dilatation (functional) • Marfan's • SLE
Presentation	• SOB & fatigue • Pulmonary oedema / haemoptysis • RHF (late)	• SOB & fatigue • Other LVF (orthopnoea, PND)
Features [↕] — T	• Mid-diastolic	• Pansystolic
I	• 1–4	• 1–6
P	• Apex	• Apex
P	• On LHS & expiration (bell)	• –
Q	• Rumbling (low-pitched)	• Blowing
R	• None	• Axilla
S	• Opening snap • Tapping apex • AF • Loud 1st heart sound • Mitral facies • Signs of RHF	• 3rd heart sound • Thrusting, displaced apex • Quiet 1st heart sound • Obliterated 2nd heart sound • AF • Audible 'click' in valve prolapse
ECG features	• AF common • P mitrale (bifid P waves)	• AF common • VEBs
CXR features	• Enlarged left atrium • Pulmonary venous congestion	• Cardiomegaly (late) • Cardiac failure [p5]

ΔΔ	• Austin Flint (2° AR)
	• Carey Coombs (rheumatic fever)
	• TS (usually rheumatic)
		• VSD (important ΔΔ post-MI)
		• TR (usually functional)
		  ○ Pulsatile hepatomegaly
		  ○ Giant V waves in JVP
		• AS (in ΔΔ for any systolic murmur)

Medical Rx	• AF Rx + anticoagulation • Diuretics	• AF Rx + anticoagulation • Diuretics • ACEi (HTN worsens MR)

Indications for surgery	• Valvuloplasty
	  ○ More than mild disease
	• Valve replacement / repair
	  ○ Associated MR
	  ○ Rigid, calcified valve
	  ○ Persistent LA thrombus
		• More than mild disease
		• Evidence of LV dysfunction
		• **Do not delay until irreversible structural damage**

2. HEART MURMURS

	Aortic stenosis	Aortic regurgitation
Aetiology	• Rheumatic heart disease • Calcified bicuspid valve (age 50–60) • Calcified tricuspid valve (age 70+)	• Rheumatic heart disease • IE • Luetic heart disease (syphilis) • Bicuspid valve • Hypertension • Aortic dissection • Marfan's • RA • Ankylosing spondylitis
Presentation	1. SOB 2. Syncope } Classic OSCE question 3. Angina	• SOB & fatigue • Palpitations • (Often asymptomatic)
Features [⇨] **T**	• Ejection systolic	• Early diastolic
I	• 1–6	• 1–4
P	• Aortic	• LSE
P	• –	• Sitting up & expiration (diaphragm)
Q	• Crescendo–decrescendo	• Breath-like (high-pitched)
R	• Carotids	• None
S	• 4th heart sound • Heaving apex • Slow-rising pulse • Narrow pulse pressure • Ejection click • Quiet 2nd heart sound (if severe)	• 3rd heart sound • Thrusting, displaced apex • Collapsing pulse • Wide pulse pressure • Eponymous signs [⇨] • Austin Flint murmur (mid-diastolic)
ECG features	• LVH / LV strain pattern	–
CXR features	–	• Cardiomegaly • Cardiac failure [p4]
ΔΔ	• Aortic sclerosis [⇨] • HOCM • PS (usually congenital) • MR (in ΔΔ for any systolic murmur)	• PR • Graham Steele (PR 2° pulmonary hypertension)
Medical Rx	–	• Diuretics • Vasodilators
Indications for surgery	• Symptomatic (prognosis 3 years) • Asymptomatic with gradient > 50 mmHg (controversial) • Valvuloplasty if unfit for surgery	• More than mild disease • **Do not delay until irreversible structural damage**

System for describing features of a heart murmur

It can be difficult to recall the features of a murmur. To help do this, use a method such as the TIPPQRS system. Keep reciting T-I-P-P-Q-R-S to yourself until it comes instantly.

T   Timing
I   Intensity – thrills are rare so say grade 2 if quiet and grade 3 if loud (don't say grade 1 & claim to be an expert!)
P_1 Position of stethoscope on precordium where heard loudest
P_2 Position of pt when murmur heard loudest – usually only relevant to diastolic murmurs
Q   Quality
R   Radiation
S   Systemic features – other heart sounds, characteristics of the apex beat / pulse, etc.

How to present your findings

Go through TIPPQRS

- On auscultation, the 1st and 2nd heart sounds are normal (or loud / quiet / prosthetic / not heard)
- There is a ⎡T⎤ murmur of grade ⎡I⎤ intensity heard loudest in the ⎡P_1⎤ area with the pt ⎡P_2⎤
- The murmur is ⎡Q⎤ in nature and radiates to the ⎡R⎤ (or does not radiate)
- There is an associated ⎡S⎤ (3rd/4th heart sounds, apex beat & pulse characteristics, etc.)
- In summary my findings on examination fit with a diagnosis of _____
- List the differential diagnosis if appropriate
- If native valves: there are no stigmata of IE or signs of heart failure (if you have checked!)
- If prosthetic valve: there is no evidence of valve failure or IE

Example 1: On auscultation, the 1st and 2nd heart sounds are normal. There is an early diastolic murmur of grade 2 intensity heard loudest at the lower left sternal edge with the pt sitting forward and breath held in expiration. The murmur is high-pitched and breath-like in nature and does not radiate. There is an associated 3rd heart sound, a thrusting apex beat and a collapsing pulse. In summary, my findings on examination fit with a diagnosis of aortic regurgitation. There are no apparent stigmata of infective endocarditis or signs of heart failure.

Example 2: On auscultation, a normal 1st heart sound is audible with a prosthetic 2nd heart sound. There is an associated ejection systolic murmur of grade 3 intensity heard loudest in the aortic area. The murmur has a crescendo–decrescendo quality and radiates to both carotids. This is likely to be a flow murmur across a prosthetic aortic valve. There is no evidence of valvular complication, particularly valve failure or IE.

NOTES

By far the most common murmurs in OSCEs are AS and MR, but AR does pop up pretty frequently so *always* palpate the carotid pulse when auscultating and decide if the murmur occurs with the pulse (i.e. systolic) or between pulses (i.e. diastolic). Remember left-sided murmurs are louder on expiration, right-sided murmurs on inspiration.

Grading of murmur intensity
- Grade 1 Very faint, just audible by an expert in optimal conditions
- Grade 2 Quiet, just audible by a non-expert in optimal conditions
- Grade 3 Moderately loud
- Grade 4 Loud with palpable thrill
- Grade 5 Very loud with thrill, audible with stethoscope partly off chest   } Systolic only
- Grade 6 Very loud with thrill, audible without a stethoscope

Stigmata of infective endocarditis
- Changing heart murmurs
- Finger clubbing
- Splinter haemorrhages
- Mild splenomegaly
- Microscopic haematuria
- Eponymous signs (rare!)
  - Osler's nodes on finger pulps
  - Janeway lesions on palms and soles
  - Roth spots on the retina

Complications of prosthetic valves
- Structural valve failure*
- Paravalvular leak*
- Thrombosis & obstruction
- Infective endocarditis
- Intravascular haemolysis
- (Warfarin-related complications)

*Both cause regurgitant murmurs

Aortic 'sclerosis'
- *Asymptomatic*
- Does not radiate to carotids
- No slow-rising pulse
- Normal pulse pressure
- 2nd heart sound normal / loud

Eponymous signs in AR
- Corrigan's: Exaggerated carotid pulse
- Quinke's: Nailbed pulsation
- De Musset's: Head-nodding
- Duroziez's: Diastolic femoral murmur
- Traube's: 'Pistol shot' femorals

Indications for a bioprosthetic valve (do not require warfarinisation but only last 10–15 years)
1. Elderly
   (if you predict that valve will outlast pt)
2. Contraindication to warfarin
   (e.g. Woman of childbearing age – considered on a case-by-case basis, weighing up against need to re-replace valve in future)

	Action / Examine for	ΔΔ / Potential findings / Extra information
Introduction	• Wash hands • Introduce yourself, explain examination & gain consent • Expose & position pt (top off, supine at 45°)	 → If only examining posterior chest, sit on side of bed now
End of bed	• Appearance – unwell / distressed / dyspnoeic / in pain • Accessory muscle use, pursed-lip breathing • Nutritional status / cachexia • Oxygen, fluids and medications • *Look* inside sputum pot if available	 → Pursed lip breathing = airway obstruction (usually COPD) → COPD, malignancy → Inhalers & nebulisers especially → Describe colour, purulence, presence of blood, etc.
Hands	• Peripheral cyanosis • Feel temperature • Dilated veins • Tar staining / coal dust tattoos • 1st web space wasting	→ PVD, Raynaud's, CCF or with central cyanosis [p4] → Central cyanosis = warm, pure peripheral cyanosis = cold [p4] → Hypercapnia → Smoking / mining (risk of coal-worker's pneumoconiosis) → T_1 lesion (e.g. Pancoast tumour)
Nails	• Finger clubbing (look carefully) • Koilonychia	→ Ca, ILD, suppurative lung disease, etc. [p112] → Iron deficiency anaemia (cause of SOB)

Wrist	• Flapping tremor (asterixis)
	• Fine physiological tremor
	• Respiratory rate
	• Radial pulse
	  ○ Rate
	  ○ Volume
		→ Respiratory failure (CO_2 retention), hepatic / renal failure
		→ β_2-agonist Rx (e.g. Salbutamol)
		→ Count over 15 sec whilst pretending to take pulse
		
		→ Tachycardia if unwell, distressed, on β_2-agonist Rx
		→ Bounding in hypercapnia

Face	• Cushingoid (moon face, plethora, acne, hirsute)	→ Long-term steroid Rx (e.g. for CFA), others [p53]
Eyes	• Conjunctival pallor • Horner's (ptosis, miosis)	→ Anaemia (cause of SOB) → Pancoast tumour [⇨]
Mouth	• Central cyanosis • Candida	→ Hypoxic lung disease, cardiac shunt, abnormal Hb [p4] → Steroid inhalers, immunocompromised pt

Neck	• JVP [p3 for technique]
	• Trachea
	  ○ "I'm going to feel for your windpipe"
	  ○ Position
	  ○ Cricosternal distance
	  ○ "Take a deep breath in"
	  ○ Tug on inspiration
	• Lymph nodes
	  ○ "Do you have any pain in your neck?"
	  ○ Palpate systematically [p110 for technique]
		→ Elevated in RHF, PE, SVC obstruction, etc. [p4]
		
		→ Deviates towards collapse, away from tension / big effusion
		→ Normally 2–3 fingers, reduced in hyperinflation (COPD)
		
		→ Hyperinflation (COPD)
		
		→ Tender = infection, non-tender = suspicious of malignancy

The chest – Anterior chest with pt supine at 45°, then repeat on posterior chest with pt sitting on side of bed, arms crossed in front to separate scapulae

Inspection	• A–P diameter	→ Hyperinflation (COPD)
	• Scars (check carefully around the sides & back)	→ Thoracotomy (lobectomy / pneumonectomy), old chest drain sites
	• Deformity of chest / spine	→ Pectus excavatum, pectus carinatum (asthma), scoliosis
	• Intercostal indrawing (*Hoover's sign*)	→ Hyperinflation (COPD)
Palpation	• Chest expansion	
	○ *"Take deep breaths in and out"*	
	○ Watch chest wall movement first	→ Large degree of asymmetry may be obvious on inspection
	○ Palpate chest wall in 2 separate places	→ Assess symmetry *only*, not degree of expansion
	• Apex beat (particularly lateral / medial displacement)	→ Mediastinal shift (collapse, tension, big effusion)
	• RV heave	→ RVH (possible cor pulmonale)
Percussion	• Assess percussion note	→ Resonant, dull, stony dull [⇨]
	○ Start in supraclavicular fossae & work down chest	→ 8–10 places is usually sufficient
	○ Compare side to side, including axillae	
	○ Map out any abnormalities	
Auscultation (Diaphragm unless very hairy or skinny)	• Breath sounds & added noises	→ [⇨]
	○ *"Take deep breaths in and out through your mouth"*	
	○ Same sequence as for percussion	→ 8–10 places is usually sufficient
	○ Listen for breath sound presence & character	→ Character can be vesicular or bronchial (consolidation)
	○ Wheeze	→ Small airway obstruction (asthma, COPD)
	○ Crepitations	→ Fluid in airspaces: secretions, pus, oedema
	○ If crepitations heard, ask pt to cough & listen again	→ If due to normal secretions, crepitations should clear with cough
	• Vocal resonance	→ ↑ in consolidation, ↓ in collapse / effusion / pneumothorax
	○ *"Say 99 each time I put my stethoscope on your chest"*	
	○ Same sequence as for percussion	→ 8–10 places is usually sufficient
	• Whispering pectoriloquy	→ Loud conduction of whispered voice due to consolidation
	○ *"Now whisper 99 each time I touch your chest"*	
	○ Check only in areas of ↑ VR or bronchial breathing	

Back	• Sacral oedema	→ RHF
Ankles	• Peripheral oedema	→ RHF (e.g. cor pulmonale), multiple other causes [p113]

Concluding remarks	• See sputum pot (if not already seen)
	• Observation chart (BP, temperature, SaO$_2$)
	• Investigations: Peak flow, PFTs, CXR, ABG

How to present your findings

Work through the examination sequence
- The pt was [dyspnoeic / comfortable] at rest breathing [air / O₂], and [cyanosed / not cyanosed]
- The respiratory rate was ___ breaths per min
- Always comment on clubbing, lymphadenopathy and mediastinal shift
- List any other peripheral signs found
- Comment on expansion, percussion, breath sounds, added sounds, vocal resonance
- Give differential diagnosis
- Comment on the presence / absence of cor pulmonale if chronic lung disease (COPD, ILD)

Example: The pt was dyspnoeic at rest breathing air, and centrally cyanosed. The respiratory rate was 25 breaths per min. There was finger clubbing but no lymphadenopathy or mediastinal shift. Chest expansion was symmetrical and the percussion note resonant throughout. Breath sounds were present throughout the chest and vesicular. In addition fine inspiratory crepitations were heard bibasally. Vocal resonance was normal. The differential diagnosis includes interstitial lung disease and pulmonary oedema.

	Consolidation	Collapse	Effusion*	Pneumothorax	Pneumonectomy
Mediastinal shift	–	Towards	Away if big	Away if tension	Towards
Percussion note	Dull	Dull	Stony dull	(Hyper) resonant	Dull
Breath sounds	Bronchial or ↓	↓ or absent	↓ or absent	↓ or absent	Absent
Vocal resonance	↑	↓ or absent	↓ or absent	↓ or absent	Absent

Lobectomy / pneumonectomy
- Given away by thoracotomy scar on chest, but some examiners will hide this to test you
- Indications: Bronchogenic Ca (25% of non-SCLC is resectable), bronchiectasis, trauma, TB

*Raised hemidiaphragm
- Examination findings identical to effusion
- CXR to differentiate
- Due to phrenic nerve palsy
- Caused by thoracic surgery / trauma / malignancy

Signs of hyperinflation
- Reduced cricosternal distance ± tracheal tug
- Increased A–P diameter
- Intercostal indrawing (Hoover's sign)
- Apex beat not palpable
- Hyper-resonant percussion note

NOTES

ΔΔ Interstitial lung disease (pulmonary fibrosis)
1. Idiopathic
   - Cryptogenic fibrosing alveolitis
2. Due to inhaled antigen (i.e. EAA)
   - Bird fancier's lung
   - Farmer's lung
3. Due to inhaled irritant
   - Asbestosis
   - Silicosis
   - Coal worker's pneumoconiosis
4. Associated with systemic disease
   - SLE
   - RA
   - Sarcoid
   - Systemic sclerosis
5. Drug-induced
   - Methotrexate
   - Amiodarone

ΔΔ Horner's syndrome
- Central lesion
  - Stroke / tumour / MS
  - Syringobulbia
- T_1 root lesion
  - Spondylosis
  - Neurofibroma
- Brachial plexus lesion
  - Pancoast tumour
  - Cervical rib
  - Trauma / birth injury (Klumpke's)
- Neck lesion
  - Tumour
  - Carotid artery aneurysm
  - Sympathectomy
- With cluster headaches

Features of bronchial breathing
- Loud and blowing
- Length of inspiration = expiration
- Audible gap between inspiration & expiration
- Reproducible by placing your stethoscope over your own trachea and listening

ΔΔ Bibasal crepitations
- Fine
  - Pulmonary oedema
  - Interstitial lung disease
- Coarse
  - Bronchiectesis
  - Cystic fibrosis
  - Bibasal pneumonia

ΔΔ Pleural effusion
- Transudate (Protein <30 g/l)
  - LVF
  - Volume overload
  - Hypoalbuminaemia [p113]
  - Meig's syndrome
- Exudate (protein >30 g/l)
  - Infection
    - pneumonia
    - TB
  - Infarction
    - PE
  - Inflammation
    - RA
    - SLE
  - Malignancy
    - bronchogenic
    - mesothelioma

NOTES

Action / Examine for	ΔΔ / Potential findings / Extra information
Introduction • Wash hands • Introduce yourself, explain examination & gain consent • Expose pt (xiphisternum to pubic symphysis) • Position pt (supine at 45º) • *"Do you have any pain in your tummy? If so, where?"*	 → Traditional 'nipples to knees' exposure is rarely necessary → Do not lie flat yet
End of bed • Appearance – unwell / distressed / in pain • Oxygen, drips, catheters, medications, drains • Nutritional status / cachexia	 → Wasting due to malabsorption or synthetic liver failure
Hands • Tendon xanthomata • Dupuytren's contracture – *feel* palm for this • Palmar erythema	→ Hyperlipidaemia (PBC, cholestasis) → CLD, diabetes, heavy labour, phenytoin, trauma, familial → CLD, pregnancy, hyperthyroidism, RA
Nails • Finger clubbing (look carefully) • Leuconychia • Koilonychia	→ IBD, cirrhosis, lymphoma, coeliac disease, etc. [p112] → Hypoalbuminaemia (CLD, other causes) [p112] → Iron-deficiency anaemia (e.g. GI bleeding)
Wrist • Flapping tremor (*asterixis*) • Radial pulse rate – palpate briefly	→ Hepatic failure (encephalopathy), respiratory / renal failure → Quick assessment of circulatory status
Arms • Bruising • IVDU marks	→ CLD (due to thombocytopaenia, clotting factors, falls) → Risk of hepatitis B & C
Face • Cushingoid (moon face, plethora, acne, hirsute) • Parotid enlargement (*sialoadenosis*)	→ Alcohol excess (alcoholic pseudo-Cushing's), others [p53] → Alcohol excess
Eyes • Scleral icterus • Corneal arcus & xanthelasma • Episcleritis / conjunctivitis • Conjunctival pallor	→ Jaundice (implies serum bilirubin >35 µmol/l) → Hyperlipidaemia (PBC, cholestasis) → Associated with IBD [⇨] → Anaemia
Mouth • Angular stomatitis & glossitis (large, smooth tongue) • Oral candidiasis • Apthous ulcers • Fetor hepaticus (musty, sweet breath odour)	→ Iron / folate / B_{12} deficiency → Immunodeficiency → IBD (especially Crohn's) → Hepatic failure (mercaptan accumulation)

Neck
 • Lymph nodes
    ○ *"Do you have any pain in your neck?"*
    ○ Palpate systematically [p111 for technique]
	
	 → Virchow's node = left supraclavicular (e.g. gastric Ca)

Chest / Back • Gynaecomastia • Loss of secondary sexual hair • Spider naevi – *depress* to demonstrate central filling	→ CLD, drugs, testicular failure, etc. [⇨] → CLD → Occur in distribution of SVC. ≥5 suggests CLD.

The abdomen – Lie flat with one pillow & arms resting at sides to relax musculature		
Inspection	• Abdominal distension	→ The 6 Fs: **F**at, **F**luid, **F**latus, **F**aeces, **F**etus, **F**lipping big masses
	• Caput medusa (dilated veins from umbilicus outwards)	→ Portal hypertension
	• Scars	→ Numerous types [⇨]
Palpation (and a little percussion)	• General palpation	→ Tenderness, guarding, masses
	○ Get down on one knee, keep watching pt's face	→ Watching the face is key; examiners will scrutinise you for it
	○ *"Tell me if I cause you any discomfort"*	
	○ Start furthest away from any tender area	
	○ Work round 9 areas, light then deep palpation	→ Keep watching the pt's face!
	• Liver	→ Hepatomegaly [⇨]
	○ *"Take deep breaths in and out"*	
	○ Start in RIF, work up towards right costal margin	
	○ Feel for liver edge during *inspiration*	→ Liver edge will flick under your fingers as it descends
	○ Percuss out upper & lower hepatic borders	→ Percuss down from axilla in ♀ to find upper border
	• Spleen	→ Splenomegaly [⇨]
	○ *"Take deep breaths in and out"*	→ [p20: differentiating between spleen & left kidney]
	○ Start in RIF, work up towards left costal margin	→ As for liver, feel during inspiration
	○ If not felt, repeat with pt on RHS and your left hand gently pulling pt's left lower ribs forward	→ Encourages an enlarged spleen to come out from behind ribs
	• Kidneys – ballot each in turn	→ [p20: ΔΔ unilateral / bilateral enlarged kidneys]
	• AAA – palpate deeply with 2 hands above umbilicus	→ Do this *very* briefly unless specifically instructed – not technically GI but cause of abdominal symptoms
Percussion	• Shifting dullness	→ Ascites (≥1.5 l of fluid present if shifting dullness) [⇨]
	○ Percuss away from midline towards left flank	→ Avoids hepatic dullness on the right
	○ Leave finger at first point of dullness	
	○ Roll pt towards you	
	○ Percuss again – if now tympanic test is +ve	→ Fluid (& dullness) shifts with gravity
Auscultation	• Bowel sounds – just below umbilicus (1 min max)	→ Active, sluggish, tinkling / obstructive
	• Renal bruits – superior and lateral to umbilicus	→ Renal artery disease
	• Liver bruit if liver edge felt	→ HCC, AV malformation, TIPSS

Legs	• Peripheral oedema	→ CLD, multiple other causes [p113]
	• Erythema nodosum	→ IBD [p103 for ΔΔ]
	• Pyoderma gangrenosum	→ IBD, RA

Concluding remarks	• Examine groins, genitalia & perform PR exam	→ Groin herniae, testicular atrophy in CLD
	• Observation chart (BP, temperature, SaO$_2$)	

15 (left margin, bottom)

Abdominal scars
1. Kocher's (subcostal) – open cholecystectomy
2. Right paramedian laparotomy – various (e.g. pancreatic transplant)
3. Midline laparotomy
4. Nephrectomy
5. Gridiron – appendicectomy
6. Laparoscopic – various (cholecystectomy, appendectomy, gynae procedures)
7. Left paramedian – anterior resection of rectum
8. Pfannenstiel / transverse suprapubic – TAH, Caesarian section

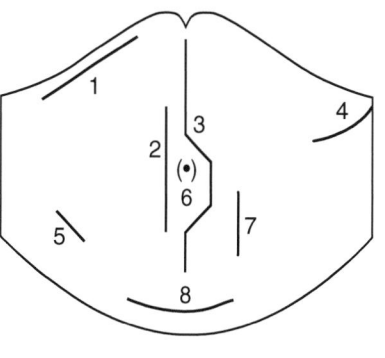

Multifactorial aetiology of ascites in CLD
1. Portal hypertension
2. Hypoalbuminaemia
3. Salt & water retention 2° RAAS activation

ΔΔ Ascites – compare with ΔΔ pleural effusion
- Transudate (protein <30 g/l)
  - CLD (75% of ascites)
  - RHF
  - Volume overload
  - Hypoalbuminaemia [p113]
  - Constrictive pericarditis
- Exudate (protein >30 g/l)
  - Infection
    - SBP
    - TB
  - Inflammation
    - pancreatitis
  - Malignancy
    - luminal (stomach / colon)
    - pancreas
    - liver (primary / metastatic)
    - ovarian
    - lymphoma

ΔΔ Hepatomegaly
Remember the categories: 2 Is, 2 Bs & 2 Cs
- Infection
  - Viral hepatitis*
  - EBV*
  - Malaria*
  - Hepatic abscess
- Infiltration
  - Sarcoid*
  - Amyloid*
  - Fatty liver
  - Haemochromatosis
- Blood-related
  - Lymphoma*
  - Leukaemia*
  - Myeloproliferative disorders*
  - Haemolytic anaemias*
- Biliary
  - PBC
  - PSC
- Cancer
  - Primary HCC
  - Metastatic deposits
- Congestion
  - RHF
  - Tricuspid regurgitation
  - Budd–Chiari syndrome

*Important causes of hepatosplenomegaly – a tricky list which you need to learn

NOTES

Extra-intestinal manifestations of IBD
- Finger clubbing
- Mouth ulcers (especially Crohn's)
- Eyes:
  - Episcleritis
  - Conjunctivitis
- Skin:
  - Erythema nodosum
  - Pyoderma gangrenosum
- Joints: Seronegative spondyloarthropathy
- PSC (especially UC)
- Amyloidosis (especially Crohn's)

ΔΔ Gynaecomastia
- Physiological (puberty / elderly)
- Testicular failure
  - Klinefelter's syndrome
  - Viral orchitis / testicular trauma
  - Haemodialysis
- Increased oestrogen
  - Chronic liver disease
  - Thyrotoxicosis
  - Oestrogen-secreting tumour
- Drug-induced (e.g. digoxin, isoniazid, spiro)

Liver edge characteristics
- Smooth
  - Venous congestion
  - Fatty infiltration
- Knobbly
  - Metastases
  - Cysts
- Pulsatile
  - Tricuspid regurgitation
- Tender
  - Hepatitis
  - RHF (capsular pain)
- Bruit
  - HCC
  - AV malformation
  - TIPSS

Causes of Massive splenomegaly (past umbilicus)
- Malaria
- Myelofibrosis
- CML

Other important causes of splenomegaly
- Infective endocarditis
- RA (if low WCC this is Felty's syndrome)

A note on portal hypertension
- Does not *cause* hepatomegaly
- Does cause splenomegaly
- When associated with early hepatic disease (e.g. chronic active hepatitis) which itself causes hepatomegaly, the overall result may be hepatosplenomegaly
- When associated with relatively late hepatic disease (e.g. cirrhosis) which causes a shrunken liver, the overall result is isolated splenomegaly
- Also causes caput medusae, oesophageal varices, gastropathy & ascites

NOTES

Action / Examine for	ΔΔ / Potential findings / Extra information
Introduction • Wash hands • Introduce yourself, explain examination & gain consent • Expose pt (xiphisternum to pubic symphysis) • Position pt (supine at 45°) • *"Do you have any pain in your tummy? If so, where?"*	 → Traditional 'nipples to knees' exposure is rarely necessary → Do not lie flat yet
End of bed • Appearance – unwell / distressed / in pain • Oxygen, drips, catheters, medications, drains • Nutritional status / cachexia	
Wrists • Flapping tremor (*asterixis*) • Radial pulse rate – palpate briefly	 → Renal failure, hepatic / respiratory failure → Quick assessment of circulatory status

Arms
 • Look for AV fistula
   ○ Wrist
   ○ Antecubital fossa
 • Examine AV fistula if present
   ○ Palpate for thrill
   ○ Auscultate for loud bruit
 • Parathyroid implantation scar
   ○ Wrist
   ○ Shoulder
 • *"I would now measure BP"*
	
	 → Radio-cephalic ('Cimino') fistula
	 → Brachio-cephalic or brachio-basilic fistula
	 → You may be asked to examine this as a 'lump' [p100]
	 → Due to turbulent flow – absent if fistula thrombosed
	 → As above
	 → Parathyroid tissue implanted following parathyroidectomy
	
	 → Never measure BP on fistula arm

Face / Eyes • Conjunctival pallor • Yellow tinge to skin	 → Anaemia (common in CRF: chronic disease, epo deficiency) → Uraemia (ΔΔ jaundice)

Neck
 • JVP [p3 for technique]
 • Central venous catheter
   ○ Current
   ○ Scar from previous CV catheter at base of neck
 • Parathyroidectomy scar
	
	 → Fluid overload
	
	 → Usually a transverse scar on lower neck

The abdomen – Lie flat with one pillow & arms resting at sides to relax musculature		

Inspection	• Abdominal distension
	• Tenckhoff catheter (peritoneal dialysis)
	  ○ Current
	  ○ Scar from previous near umbilicus
	• Nephrectomy scars
	• Renal transplant scars
		→ The 6 Fs: **F**at, **F**luid, **F**latus, **F**aeces, **F**etus, **F**lipping big masses (including polycystic kidneys)
		
		→ Check flanks
		→ Right / left iliac fossa (unless pt is Jonah Lomu), *look very carefully*

Palpation	• General palpation
	  ○ Get down on one knee, keep watching pt's face
	  ○ *"Tell me if I cause you any discomfort"*
	  ○ Start furthest away from any tender area
	  ○ Work round 9 areas, light then deep palpation
	• Kidneys
	  ○ Ballot flanks for each kidney in turn
	  ○ Differentiate left kidney from spleen if necessary
	• Transplanted kidney
	  ○ Palpate for this under LIF/RIF scar
	• Liver
	  ○ Palpate if kidneys enlarged [p15 for technique]
		→ Tenderness, guarding, masses
		→ Watching the face is key; examiners will scrutinise you for it
		
		→ Keep watching the pt's face!
		→ Unilateral / bilateral enlargement [⇨]
		
		→ [⇨]
		
		→ Sometimes difficult to palpate
		
		→ Polycystic hepatomegaly can occur in APKD

Percussion	• Shifting dullness if Tenckhoff catheter *in situ*
	  ○ Percuss away from midline towards left flank
	  ○ Leave finger at first point of dullness
	  ○ Roll pt towards you
	  ○ Percuss again – if now tympanic test is +ve
		→ Ascites (in this case peritoneal dialysate)
		→ Avoids hepatic dullness on the right
		
		→ Fluid (& dullness) shifts with gravity

Auscultation	• Renal bruits – superior and lateral to umbilicus	→ Renal artery disease
Back	• Auscultate lung bases for crepitations • Palpate for sacral oedema	→ Fluid overload → Fluid overload
Ankles	• Ankle oedema	→ Fluid overload [p113]
Concluding remarks	• Observation chart (BP, temperature, SaO$_2$) • Dip urine	→ May shed light on aetiology of CRF

ΔΔ LIF mass
- Renal transplant
- Loaded colon
- Diverticular mass
- Colorectal carcinoma
- Ovarian

ΔΔ Bilateral enlarged kidneys
- APKD
- Bilateral hydronephrosis
- Amyloidosis

ΔΔ Unilateral enlarged kidney
- Hydronephrosis
- Renal cancer
- Renal cyst

ΔΔ RIF mass
- Renal transplant
- Appendix mass
- Crohn's disease (inflamed, matted small intestine)
- Caecal carcinoma
- Ovarian

Spleen versus left kidney on examination
- You can get your hand over a kidney
- Percussion note is resonant over a kidney
- Kidney is balottable
- Spleen has a notch
- Spleen moves more on respiration

Indications for dialysis in CRF
- Progressive decline in renal function (usually CKD Stage 5 = GFR <15 ml/min)
- Symptomatic uraemia despite conservative Rx
- Renal bone disease
- Pericarditis
- Volume overload despite fluid restriction & diuretics
- Hyperkalaemia despite Rx

NOTES

Components of renal bone disease
1. Osteomalacia due to vitamin D deficiency
2. Hyperparathyroidism due to ↑ serum phosphate
   - Subperiosteal bone resorption, especially on hand X-ray
   - Pepper pot skull (ΔΔ multiple myeloma)
3. Osteosclerosis due to prolonged hyperparathyroidism
   - 'Rugger jersey' spine
4. Osteoporosis

Complications of haemodialysis
- Hypotension
- Hypovolaemia
- Hypokalaemia
- Disequilibration syndrome (cerebral oedema)
- Dialysis-related amyloidosis (β_2-microglobulin accumulation causing peripheral neuropathy, etc.)

Side-effects of post-transplant immunosuppressive drug therapy
- High-dose corticosteroids [p50]
  - Cushingoid facies (moon face, plethora, acne, hirsute)
  - Thin skin
  - Bruising
  - Abdominal obesity
  - Purple striae
  - Muscle wasting in limbs
- Ciclosporin
  - Gingival hypertrophy
  - Warty skin lesions
  - Hypertrichosis (werewolf syndrome)

NOTES

Introduction	• Wash hands • Introduce yourself, explain examination & gain consent • Position pt (sitting opposite you, 1–2 m away with your heads at roughly the same level)

	Attribute	Method of examination	ΔΔ / Potential findings / Extra information
I Olfactory	**Smell**	• *"Have you noticed any changes in your sense of smell?"*	
II Optic	**Visual acuity**	• *"Do you wear glasses or contact lenses?"* • *"Have you had any problems with your vision recently?"* • Ask pt to read something, *covering one eye at a time* • Indicate you would ideally use a Snellen chart at 6 m	→ A common mistake is to allow pt to use both eyes at once

	Visual fields	• Inattention
		  ○ *"Look at my nose"*
		  ○ Put your arms directly out to sides, pointing fingers
		  ○ *"Keep looking at my nose; point to the finger I move"*
		  ○ Wiggle left, right, then both fingers at once
		• Visual fields (ideally use white hat pin)
		  ○ *"Look at my nose; can you see my whole face?"*
		  ○ Ask pt to cover left eye with left hand
		  ○ *"With your right eye, look into my left eye"*
		  ○ Close / cover your own right eye
		  ○ *"Keep looking into my eye and tell me when you see the white dot out of the corner of your eye"*
		  ○ Move hat pin towards centre from 4 corners of visual field
		  ○ Compare pt's visual fields with your own
		  ○ Repeat on pt's right eye
			→ Usually the result of a stroke
			
			→ Pt with visual inattention will only see one finger move
			→ Crude assessment of fields
			
			→ Simply closing your eye frees both your arms to slickly manoeuvre the hat pin
			
			→ Top left, bottom left, top right, bottom right

	Pupillary reflexes
	(also CN III)
		• Ask pt to concentrate on a spot on the wall
		• *"I am going to briefly shine my torch into your eyes"*
		• Look for direct & consensual responses
		• Swinging torch test
		  ○ Repeatedly 'swing' torch between eyes
		  ○ Look for inappropriate pupillary dilation when light shone at that eye
			→ RAPD (Marcus Gunn pupil)
			→ Shine in left eye for 1 sec, right eye for 1 sec & keep repeating

	Fundus	• *"Ideally I would like to examine the fundus by ophthalmoscopy"*	

| III Oculomotor IV Trochlear VI Abducens | Eye movements | • Note any ptosis & abnormal position of eye
• *"Keep your head still and follow my finger with your eyes"*
• *"Tell me if you see double at any point"*
• Finger at least 50 cm from face, move slowly in an 'H' pattern
• Look for obvious ophthalmoplegia & nystagmus
• If suggestion of nystagmus, move finger more quickly to elicit
• If there is diplopia
  ○ Ask if images separated horizontally or vertically
  ○ Cover each eye in turn, which image disappears?
  ○ Looking to side – lateral image from affected eye
  ○ Looking down – lower image from affected eye
  ○ Looking up – upper image from affected eye | → CN III palsy: ptosis

→ This is essential

→ Slight nystagmus at extremes of lateral gaze occurs in some normal individuals
→ Should allow identification of ophthalmoplegic eye though can be difficult for pt |
| | Accommodation | • *"Keep looking at my finger"*
• Move finger slowly in towards pt's nose
• Check that pupils constrict appropriately during convergence | → Note that convergence is preserved in INO [p28] |

V Trigeminal	Sensory	• Ask pt to close eyes
		• *"Say 'yes' when you feel me touching your face"*
		• Move from side to side: *"Does it feel the same on both sides?"*
		  ○ Ophthalmic division: above eyebrows
		  ○ Maxillary division: over zygoma
		  ○ Mandibular division: chin either side of the midline
			→ You could assess pain (neurotip) and light touch (cotton wool) sensation here if time

	Motor	• Jaw opening against resistance
		  ○ Push upwards on bottom of pt's chin
		  ○ *"Open your jaw against my hand"*
		  ○ Jaw will deviate towards side of weakness
		• Jaw clenching
		  ○ Palpate for masseter contraction above angle of jaw
			→ Pterygoid muscles
			
			→ Masseter muscles

	Reflexes	• Corneal reflex
		  ○ Can be assessed indirectly
		  ○ Test sensation inside nostrils with wisp of cotton wool
		• Jaw jerk
		  ○ *"Let your mouth hang open"*
		  ○ Place your thumb on pt's chin
		  ○ Strike thumb briskly with tendon hammer
		    ▪ Minimal / absent = normal
		    ▪ Brisk = UMN lesion
			→ Same branch of trigeminal is implicated in nostril sensation and corneal reflex
			
			→ Stroke / tumour / MS, etc.

	Attribute	Method of examination	ΔΔ / Potential findings / Extra info
VII Facial	**Facial tone**	• Look for signs of reduced facial tone 　○ Reduced wrinkling of forehead 　○ Drooping of corner of mouth 　○ Flattening of the nasolabial fold	→ Occurs in LMN facial nerve lesions only [⇨]
	Facial movements	• Raise eyebrows • Screw up eyes 　○ *"Keep them tightly shut"* – try to pull open 　○ Bell's sign = upgaze on attempted eye closure • Puff out cheeks • Show gums	→ Facial nerve (e.g. Bell's) palsy
	Other functions	• Chorda tympani – supplies anterior $^2/_3$ of tongue 　○ *"Have you noticed any change in taste?"* • Branch to stapedius 　○ *"Are you troubled by loud noises?"*	
VIII Vestibulo-cochlear	**Hearing**	• Stroke tragus or occlude external auditory meatus of one ear • Ask pt to repeat numbers you whisper in their other ear • Repeat with other ear	→ Crude assessment of hearing
	Special tests	• Rinne test 　○ Assess each ear in turn 　○ First place heel of vibrating tuning fork on mastoid process behind ear – *"This is sound number one"* 　○ Secondly place prongs of vibrating tuning fork close to (but not touching) the external auditory meatus – *"This is sound number two"* 　○ *"Which was louder, sound one or two?"* • Weber test 　○ Place heel of vibrating tuning fork in centre of pt's forehead 　○ *"Do you hear the sound more on the left or right, or just in the middle of your head?"*	→ [⇨ for interpretation] → Bone conduction → Air conduction → [⇨ for interpretation]

IX	Glosso-pharyngeal
	X Vagus
	XII Hypoglossal
		Bulbar function	• Soft palate movement
			  ○ Shine torch in mouth
			  ○ *"Say 'ahhh' please"*
			  ○ Look at movement of uvula
			  ○ Pulled *away from* side of weakness
			• Speech
			• Swallowing water
				→ Generally assessed throughout examination

		Tongue	• Appearance
			  ○ Normal
			  ○ Flaccid, wasted & fasciculating
			  ○ Spastic & contracted
			• Movements
			  ○ *"Stick your tongue straight out"*
			  ○ Deviates *towards* side of weakness
			  ○ *"Move your tongue from side to side"*
				→ Bulbar palsy [⇨]
				→ Pseudobulbar palsy [⇨]

XI	Spinal accessory	**Motor**	• Trapezius – shrug shoulders against resistance • Sternocleidomastoids – turn head against resistance	

Causes of grouped cranial nerve palsies
- Cerebellopontine angle tumour
  (acoustic neuroma or meningioma)
  - Corneal reflex lost first (V)
  - Then VII & VIII
  - Then rest of V
  - Sometimes IX & X
- Paget's disease of bone
  (bony impingement on nerves)
  - V, VII & VIII
- Gradenigo's syndrome
  (complication of otitis media)
  - V & VI
- Syringobulbia
  - Bulbar palsy (IX, X & XII)
  - VIII – vertigo & nystagmus
  - V – facial pain / sensory loss
  - VII sparing
  - May have Horner's syndrome
  - May have syringomyelia [p18]
- Cavernous sinus thrombosis
  - III, IV & VI (VI most common)
  - V – pain (especially ophthalmic division)
  - Corneal reflex may be lost (V)
  - Also headache, periorbital oedema,
    proptosis

Causes of *any* cranial nerve palsy
- Diabetes ('microangiopathy of the vasa
  nervorum')
- Stroke
- MS
- Tumour
- Sarcoid
- SLE
- Vasculitis

ΔΔ Ptosis
- Unilateral
  - CN III palsy
  - Horner's syndrome
  - Congenital
- Bilateral
  - Myasthenia gravis
  - Myotonic dystrophy
  - Congenital

Features of CN III palsy
- Eye deviated 'down and out'
- Ptosis
- Dilated pupil if complete*

NOTES

ΔΔ Specific cranial nerve palsies

- I Olfactory
  - Trauma
  - Frontal lobe tumour
  - Meningitis
- II Optic
  - Monocular blindness
    - MS
    - GCA
  - Bitemporal hemianopia
    - pituitary adenoma
    - internal carotid artery aneurysm
  - Homonymous hemianopia
    - anything behind chiasm
    - stroke / tumour / abscess
- III Oculomotor
  - Partial (pupil spared)
    - diabetes*
  - Complete
    - PCA aneurysm
    - raised ICP with tentorial herniation
- IV Trochlear
  - Single palsy rare
  - Usually due to orbit trauma
- V Trigeminal
  - Idiopathic (trigeminal neuralgia)
  - Acoustic neuroma
  - Herpes zoster
- VI Abducens
  - Skull # involving petrous temporal bone
  - Nasopharyngeal carcinoma
  - Raised ICP (false localising sign)

- VII Facial
  - LMN (forehead affected)
    - Bell's palsy
    - malignant parotid tumour
    - herpes zoster (Ramsay Hunt)
    - sarcoid (often bilateral)
  - UMN (forehead spared)
    - stroke / tumour
- VIII Vestibulocochlear
  - Excessive noise levels
  - Ménière's disease
  - Furosemide
  - Aminoglycoside antibiotics (gentamicin)
- IX / X / XII Bulbar [p29]
  - LMN (bulbar palsy)
    - MND
    - diphtheria
    - polio
    - Guillain–Barré syndrome
    - syringobulbia
  - UMN (pseudobulbar palsy)
    - motor neurone disease
    - bilateral strokes
    - MS

*In diabetic oculomotor palsy the pial vessels perfusing parasympathetic fibres are unaffected by the diabetic microangiopathy, hence the pupil is spared (and the palsy 'partial')

Extra-ocular muscles
- CN III
  - Superior rectus
  - Inferior rectus
  - Medial rectus
  - Inferior oblique
- CN IV
  - Superior oblique – 'SO4'
- CN VI
  - Lateral rectus – 'LR6'

ΔΔ Ophthalmoplegia
- Myaesthenia gravis
- Cranial nerve palsy
  - [p24]
  - Remember ↑ICP & cavernous sinus thrombosis
- Graves' disease [p86]
- Wernicke's encephalopathy (particularly failure of upgaze) [p49]
- Progressive supranuclear palsy (vertical gaze) [p44]

Internuclear ophthalmoplegia
- Disorder of conjugate lateral gaze caused by lesion in the medial longitudinal fasciculus
- Causes failure of ADduction of eye on affected side
- In a left-sided INO
  - Lateral gaze to left is normal (left eye is being *ABducted*)
  - On attempting to look to the right
    - right eye ABducts normally
    - left eye fails to ADduct and remains looking straight ahead
    - right eye consequently displays nystagmus as it attempts to compensate
- Convergence is preserved (i.e. the left eye can ADduct normally as long as the goal is not lateral gaze)

ΔΔ Internuclear ophthalmoplegia
- MS (almost always the cause in a young pt)
- Stroke
- Lyme disease and tricyclic antidepressant overdose are rare causes

SR   IO

LR6 ←→ MR

IR   SO4

'depresses the adducted eye'

Nose

NOTES

Interpretation of Rinne & Weber tests:

Rinne test	Weber test	Diagnosis
Air > bone (both ears)	Central	Normal
Bone > air (left ear)	Lateralises to left ear	Conductive hearing loss in left ear
Bone > air (left ear)*	Lateralises to right ear	Complete sensorineural deafness in left ear
Air > bone (both ears)	Lateralises to left ear	Sensorineural hearing loss in right ear

*In this interesting situation, during Rinne test, sound is conducted via the skull across to the (normal) right ear when bone conduction is tested. Nothing is heard when air conduction is tested. Therefore bone is louder than air.

Features of bulbar & pseudobulbar palsies:

	Lesion	Aetiology	Tongue appearance (use to differentiate)	Other features
Bulbar palsy	LMN	• MND** • Diphtheria • Polio • Guillain-Barré syndrome • Syringobulbia	• Flaccid • Wasted • Fasciculating	• Drooling • Dysphonia • Tremulous lips
Pseudobulbar palsy	UMN	• MND** • Bilateral strokes (e.g. internal capsule) • MS	• Spastic • Contracted	• Drooling • Dysphonia • Emotional lability

** Note MND can cause either

	Action / Examine for	ΔΔ / Potential findings / Extra information
Introduction	• Wash hands • Introduce yourself, explain examination & gain consent • Expose & position pt (top off, supine at 45°) • *"Do you have any pain, tingling or weakness in your arms or hands?"*	

Inspection	• Symmetry, muscle wasting, fasciculation
	• 'UMN posture' – shoulder ADducted, elbow flexed, wrist flexed & pronated
	• Pronator drift
	  ○ Ask pt to stretch arms out in front of them, palms facing upwards
	  ○ *"Close your eyes, and keep your arms there"*
	  ○ If hand drifts down and pronates – positive result on that side
		→ Wasting & fasciculation = LMN
		→ UMN lesion (e.g. stroke)
		
		→ Subtle UMN weakness (e.g. stroke)
		→ If pt cannot do this then you don't need to do the test (i.e. weakness is already obvious)

Tone	• Take pt's hand in 'shaking hands' grip, supporting arm at elbow • *"Let your arm go totally floppy"* • Pronate / supinate to detect supinator catch • Flex / extend wrist • Flex / extend elbow • *"Tap your knee with your other hand"* – continue to flex / extend elbow • Repeat with the other arm	 → Early sign of increased tone → 'Clasp-knife' hypertonia = UMN lesion → Synkinesis (reinforces hypertonia)
Power	• *"Are you right- or left-handed?"* • Ask pt to 'push me away' or 'pull me towards you' where possible • Assess each movement on one side then compare with the other • Grade power out of 5	→ Can influence power in arms → Isotonic testing = more sensitive → [⇨] → Not all movements need testing – these cover all roots, nerves & joints

Movement	Root	Nerve
Shoulder ABduction*	C5	Axillary
Elbow flexion	C5 / C6	Musculocutaneous
Elbow extension*	C7	Radial
Wrist extension*	C7	Radial
Finger extension*	C7	Radial
Finger flexion	C8	Median + ulnar
Thumb ABduction	T1	Median
Finger ABduction	T1	Ulnar

→ *Weak in UMN lesion

Reflexes	• Ask pt to relax and close their eyes	→ If difficulty relaxing, ask to clench teeth immediately before striking tendon

Reflex	Root
Biceps jerk	C5 / C6
Triceps jerk	C7
Supinator jerk	C5 / C6

→ Strike thumb placed on tendon
→ Strike directly
→ Strike directly

Co-ordination	• 'Piano playing' – hold hands out and wiggle fingers • Hand slapping test for dysdiadokinesis [p46] • Finger–nose test [p46]	→	Difficult in UMN lesion, Parkinson's Cerebellar ataxia Cerebellar ataxia

Sensation	• Light touch (cotton wool) then pain (neurotip)
	  ○ Ask pt to close eyes, demonstrate on their sternum (midline)
	  ○ *"Say yes when you feel me touch your skin"*
	  ○ Move from side to side – *"Does it feel the same on both sides?"*
		→	Never assess with eyes open – pt may see you touch skin and say they feel it regardless

Area	Root
Above shoulder tip	C4
Regimental badge area	C5
Tip of thumb	C6
Tip of middle finger	C7
Tip of little finger	C8
Medial mid-forearm	T1

→ [⇨ for diagram]
→ [p38 for examination of hand sensation according to peripheral nerve distribution]

• Sensory level on arms if peripheral neuropathy suspected
  ○ Tap cotton wool up arm starting at tip of middle finger
  ○ Ask pt to tell you when they feel sensation *change*
  ○ Repeat on other arm

→ 'Glove and stocking' sensory loss (e.g. diabetic neuropathy)

• Joint position sense
  ○ Use middle finger DIP joint
  ○ Immobilise middle phalanx with one hand, hold distal finger by its sides
  ○ *"Close your eyes and tell me if your finger is up, down or if you're not sure"*
  ○ Randomly move finger tip up/down & ask pt its position 3–4 times
  ○ Repeat on other arm

→ Avoid touching finger pulp as this allows touch to be used, rather than simply joint position sense

• Vibration sense
  ○ Ask pt to close eyes
  ○ *"Tell me if you feel buzzing or pushing"*
  ○ Strike tuning fork to make it vibrate
  ○ Hold heel of tuning fork to middle finger tip → radial styloid → olecranon → shoulder tip
  ○ Repeat on other arm
• (Temperature – rarely formally assessed)

→ Lost early in peripheral neuropathy

→ Crude touch may be retained though vibration sense is lost

→ No need to move proximally if vibration is perceived distally

Concluding remarks	• *"I would like to complete a full neurological examination"* • Investigations: Nerve conduction studies, imaging (CT / MRI)

Clinical features of LMN lesion, UMN lesion, extrapyramidal pathology & cerebellar lesion

NOTES

	LMN lesion	UMN lesion	Extrapyramidal [p42]	Cerebellar lesion [p46]
Tone	Normal or ↓	↑ (spastic)	↑ (rigid)	↓
Power	↓	↓	Normal	Normal
Reflexes	Reduced	Brisk	Normal	Normal
Plantars	Down	Up	Down	Down
Co-ordination	Normal	↓	↓	↓↓
Other features	Wasting Fasciculation	Clonus	Resting tremor Bradykinesia Postural instability	Intention tremor Nystagmus Cerebellar speech

Grading of power (0–5)
- 5   Normal

- 4   Reduced
  Able to move against resistance

- 3   Able to move against gravity
  Unable to move against resistance

- 2   Unable to move against gravity
  Able to move if gravity eliminated

- 1   Flicker of movement only

- 0   No movement

Suggested points for assessing sensation (C4–T1)

C4: above shoulder tip

C4

Right arm anterior view

C5: regimental badge area

C5

T3

T2

C6 / T1

T1: medial mid-forearm

C6: tip of thumb

C7 / C8

C8: tip of little finger

C7: tip of middle finger

Sensory modalities carried in the spinal cord
- Spinothalamic tracts
  - Pain
  - Temperature
  - Crude touch
- Dorsal columns
  - Vibration
  - Joint position sense
  - Fine touch

Pathology of spinal cord sensory tracts
- Spinothalamic
  - Syringomyelia
  - Anterior spinal artery occlusion
- Dorsal columns
  - Tabes dorsalis (syphilis)
  - SCDC [p37]
- Any
  - MS

Syringomyelia
- Expansion of spinal cord central canal due to CSF blockage (commonly Chiari malformation)
- Spinothalamic fibres principally affected
- Loss of pain & temperature sensation in 'cape-like' distribution over arms, shoulders & upper body
- LMN signs in upper limbs, spastic paraparesis of lower limbs
- Dorsal column signs develop as canal (syrinx) further expands
- Syringobulbia if syrinx extends into brainstem [p29]

Brachial plexus injuries at birth

	Erb's palsy	Klumpke's palsy
Part of plexus injured	Upper plexus (C5–C7)	Lower plexus (C8–T1)
Mechanism of injury	Shoulder dystocia during birth	Excessive arm traction during birth
Clinical features	Sensory loss down lateral arm 'Waiter's tip' position • Shoulder ADducted • Arm internally rotated • Forearm pronated	Sensory loss in medial forearm & hand Complete claw hand Wasting of small muscles in hand Horner's syndrome may co-exist

	Action / Examine for	ΔΔ / Potential findings / Extra information
Introduction	<ul><li>Wash hands</li><li>Introduce yourself, explain examination & gain consent</li><li>Expose & position pt (pants / shorts only, supine)</li><li>"Do you have any pain, tingling or weakness in your legs or feet?"</li></ul>	
Inspection	<ul><li>Symmetry, muscle wasting, fasciculation</li><li>'UMN posture' – hip & knee extended, foot plantarflexed & inverted</li><li>Soft tissue damage due to sensory neuropathy (especially feet)</li></ul>	→ Wasting & fasciculation = LMN → UMN lesion (e.g. stroke) → Blisters, ulcers, Charcot joints

Tone	<ul><li>"Let your leg go totally floppy"</li><li>Rock leg from side to side</li><li>Suddenly pull upwards from behind knee – if leg stays straight (and heel comes off bed) this indicates hypertonia</li><li>Suddenly pull each foot into dorsiflexion to elicit clonus (3+ beats)</li></ul>	→ Don't be too rough with the pt! → UMN lesion
Power	<ul><li>Ask pt to 'push me away' or 'pull me towards you' where possible</li><li>Assess each movement on one side then compare with the other</li><li>Grade power out of 5</li></ul><table><tr><td>Movement</td><td>Root</td></tr><tr><td>Hip flexion</td><td>L1 / L2</td></tr><tr><td>Hip extension (push heel into bed)</td><td>L5 / S1</td></tr><tr><td>Knee flexion</td><td>L5 / S1</td></tr><tr><td>Knee extension</td><td>L3 / L4</td></tr><tr><td>Ankle dorsiflexion</td><td>L4</td></tr><tr><td>Big toe extension</td><td>L5</td></tr><tr><td>Ankle plantarflexion</td><td>S1</td></tr></table>	→ 'Isotonic' testing = more sensitive → [p32]
Reflexes	<ul><li>Ask pt to relax and close their eyes</li></ul><table><tr><td>Reflex</td><td>Root</td></tr><tr><td>Knee jerk (palpate tendon first)</td><td>L3 / L4</td></tr><tr><td>Ankle jerk</td><td>S1</td></tr></table><ul><li>Plantar reflexes<ul><li>Run thumb nail up lateral side of foot, watch hallux</li><li>Up / down / equivocal</li></ul></li></ul>	→ If difficulty relaxing, ask to clench teeth immediately before you strike the tendon → Different methods – choose one you like & become slick at it → First movement of hallux counts → Up (+ve Babinski) = UMN lesion
Co-ordination	<ul><li>Heel–shin test [p47]</li></ul>	→ Cerebellar ataxia

Sensation	• Light touch (cotton wool) then pain (neurotip)
	○ Ask pt to close eyes, demonstrate on their sternum (midline) → Never assess with eyes open – pt may see you touch skin and say they feel it regardless
	○ *"Say yes when you feel me touch your skin"*
	○ Move from side to side – *"Does it feel the same on both sides?"*

Area	Root
Antero-medial upper thigh	L2
Antero-medial thigh above knee	L3
Medial mid-leg	L4
Middle of dorsum of foot	L5
Lateral sole of foot	S1

→ [⇨ for diagram]

• Sensory level on legs if peripheral neuropathy suspected → 'Glove and stocking' sensory loss (e.g. diabetic neuropathy)
  ○ Tap cotton wool up antero-medial leg starting at tip of hallux
  ○ Ask pt to tell you when they feel sensation *change*
  ○ Repeat on other leg
• Joint position sense (proprioception)
  ○ Use hallux
  ○ Immobilize first metatarsal head with one hand; hold distal digit by its sides → Avoid touching pulp of hallux as this allows touch to be used, rather than simply joint position sense
  ○ *"Close your eyes and tell me when your big toe is up, down, or if you're not sure"*
  ○ Randomly move hallux up/down & ask pt its position 3–4 times
  ○ Repeat on other foot
• Vibration sense → Lost early in peripheral neuropathy
  ○ *"Close your eyes and tell me if you feel buzzing or pushing"* → Crude touch may be retained though vibration sense is lost
  ○ Strike tuning fork to make it vibrate
  ○ Hold base of fork to pulp of hallux → medial maleolus → tibial tuberosity → ASIS → No need to move proximally if vibration is perceived distally
  ○ Repeat on other leg
• (Temperature – rarely formally assessed)

Special tests	• Romberg's test → Sensory ataxia due to proprioceptive loss [⇨]
	○ Stand pt up, feet together, facing you → May be impossible if legs very weak
	○ Hover your hands above pt's shoulders
	○ *"Now close your eyes. I will catch you if necessary"*
	○ If pt suddenly becomes very unsteady – positive test → Without visual input and with impaired proprioception pt cannot maintain balance
	○ Steady pt's shoulders and instruct to open eyes
	• Straight leg raise [p77] → L5 / S1 nerve root impingement
	• Femoral stretch test [p77] → L4 nerve root impingement

Concluding remarks	• *"I would now like to assess gait"*
	• Spastic paraparesis: examine for sensory level on thorax
	• Flaccid paraparesis: perform PR & check for saddle anaesthesia
	• Investigations: nerve conduction studies / CT head / MRI spine

Suggested points for assessing sensation (L2–S1)

Anterior left
leg & dorsum
of foot

L1

L2

L2: antero-medial upper thigh

L3

L3: antero-medial thigh just above knee

Posterior left leg
& sole of foot

L4

L4: medial mid-leg

L5

L5

L4

L5: middle of dorsum of foot

L5

S1

S1

S1: lateral sole of foot

L5

NOTES

ΔΔ **Paraparesis = Bilateral leg weakness**

- Acute & progressive – not in OSCEs
  - Acute spinal cord compression (UMN)
  - Cauda equina syndrome (LMN)
  - Guillain–Barré syndrome (LMN)
- Spastic paraparesis[1] = Bilateral UMN signs
  - Sagittal sinus lesion[2]
    - parasagittal meningioma
  - Bilateral strokes
  - Syringomyelia (with upper limb signs)
  - Cord trauma
  - Cord compression[3]
    - extradural tumour
    - disc prolapse
    - spondylosis
  - Intrinsic cord disease
    - tumour
    - vascular myelopathy
    - MS

- Flaccid paraparesis = Bilateral LMN signs
  - Polio
  - Mostly motor peripheral neuropathy
    - Guillain–Barré
    - lead poisoning
    - Charcot–Marie–Tooth
  - Mixed peripheral neuropathy[4] (see below)
- Mixed UMN & LMN signs = confusing!
  - MND[2]
  - SCDC

[1] Always look for a 'sensory level' on thorax
[2] Exclusively motor signs
[3] Look for LMN signs at level of compression
[4] There will also be marked sensory loss

ΔΔ Unilateral leg weakness
- UMN
  - Stroke
  - Tumour
  - MS
- LMN
  - Root lesion
  - Nerve lesion

ΔΔ Peripheral neuropathy
- Mostly sensory
  - Diabetes mellitus
  - Uraemia (renal failure)
- Mostly motor
  - Guillain–Barré
  - Lead poisoning
  - Charcot–Marie–Tooth
- Mixed sensory / motor
  - B12 / folate deficiency (also cause SCDC)
  - Thiamine deficiency
  - Alcohol
  - Vasculitis / SLE
  - Paraneoplastic
  - Amyloid

Positive Romberg's test (sensory ataxia)
- Dorsal column loss
  - Tabes dorsalis (syphilis)
  - SCDC
  - MS
- Sensory peripheral neuropathy

[see relevant information p32]
- Clinical features of UMN lesion, LMN lesion, extrapyramidal pathology and cerebellar lesion
- System used for grading of power
- Sensory modalities in the spinal cord

SCDC (B$_{12}$ / folate deficiency)
- Spastic paraparesis
- Upgoing plantars
- Reduced knee jerks
- Loss of ankle jerks
- Dorsal column loss
  - Loss of vibration sense
  - Loss of joint position sense
  - Sensory ataxia (+ve Romberg's)

MND can cause almost any collection of motor signs

Amyotrophic lateral sclerosis (type of MND)
- Weakness
- Wasting   } LMN signs
- Fasciculation
- Spasticity   } UMN signs
- Brisk reflexes

ΔΔ Foot drop
- Common peroneal nerve palsy
- Stroke
- L4 / L5 root lesion
- MND
- Charcot–Marie–Tooth syndrome

NOTES

Action / Examine for	ΔΔ / Potential findings / Extra information
Introduction	• Wash hands • Introduce yourself, explain examination & gain consent • Expose (hands & arms up to elbows at least) • *"Do you have any pain, tingling or weakness in your arms or hands?"*	

It is worth practising both the examination of the individual nerves on their own, as well as a combined examination working through inspection → power → sensation → special tests for all 3.

Median nerve	

Inspection	• Wasting of thenar eminence
	  ○ Pt in 'begging' position, hands together with palms up
	  ○ Compare sides
	• Carpal tunnel decompression scar (palm / wrist)
		→ Much easier to identify wasting when comparing sides

Power	• Thumb ABduction
	  ○ Palm facing upwards
	  ○ *"Pull your thumb straight up towards your nose"*
	  ○ With one finger, push thumb back towards palm
	  ○ *"Don't let me push your thumb down"*
		→ Tests ABbductor pollicis brevis [LOAF ⇨]

Sensation	• Test lateral side of index finger
	  ○ Ask pt to close eyes
	  ○ *"Say yes when you feel me touch your skin"*
	  ○ *"Does that feel normal? Is it the same on both sides?"*
		→ [⇨ Fig. 1]

Special tests	• Tinel test
	  ○ Repeatedly percuss over the carpal tunnel (ventral wrist)
	  ○ Paraesthesia in the median distribution = positive test
	• Phalen test
	  ○ Wrist held in flexion for 30–60 sec
	  ○ Paraesthesia in median distribution = positive test
		→ Carpal tunnel syndrome
		
		→ Carpal tunnel syndrome

Ulnar nerve		

Inspection	• Wasting of hypothenar eminence
	  ○ Pt in 'begging' position, hands together
	  ○ Compare sides
	• Backs of hands for wasting of interossei (especially 1st)
	• Partial claw hand
	  ○ Weak medial lumbricals – clawing of little and ring fingers
	  ○ Lateral lumbricals unaffected (median innervation)
	• Check elbows
	  ○ Scars
	  ○ Evidence of trauma / deformity
		→ Skin 'sinking' between tendons
		→ [Fig. 3]
		
		→ [LOAF ⇨]

Power	• Finger ABduction
	  ○ Palm facing downwards
	  ○ Hold digits 3–5 between your thumb and fingers
	  ○ ABduct the pt's index finger for them
	  ○ With one finger push index finger back across towards 3rd finger
	  ○ *"Don't let me push your finger in"*
		→ [⇨ Fig. 2]
		→ Testing ABduction purely in the index finger rather than across all fingers is more sensitive and looks slicker

Sensation	• Test medial side of little finger • Method as above	→ [⇨ Fig. 1]

Special tests	• Froment's sign
	  ○ Ask pt to pinch piece of paper between a *straight* thumb and index finger
	  ○ Instruct to grip paper as you pull it away
	  ○ Flexed DIP joint of thumb = positive test
		→ [⇨ Fig. 4]
		→ Long thumb flexors used to compensate for weak ADductor pollicis

Radial nerve		
Inspection	• Wrist drop • (Note: No wasting in hand – no intrinsic muscles supplied by radial nerve)	→ ΔΔ C7 radiculopathy [⇨]
Power	• Wrist extension • Finger extension	
Sensation	• Test dorsal 1st interosseous space • Method as above	→ [⇨ Fig. 1]
Special tests	–	

Concluding remarks	• *"I would like to complete a full neurological examination"* • Investigations: Nerve conduction studies	

		Median nerve	Ulnar nerve	Radial nerve
Sensory innervation		Lateral palm Thumb & lateral 2½ fingers	Medial hand (palm & dorsum) Medial 1½ fingers	Lateral dorsum of hand (no fingers)
Motor innervation		**LOAF** muscles of hand • **L**ateral 2 lumbricals • **O**pponens pollicis • **AB**ductor pollicis brevis • **F**lexor pollicis brevis	Small muscles of the hand with the exception of the LOAF muscles	Extensors • Fingers • Wrist • Elbow
Mechanism of injury		Carpal tunnel syndrome	Elbow (funny bone) trauma Hand trauma (*rare*)	Humeral shaft # Saturday night palsy*
Features of palsy	Wasting	Thenar eminence	Hypothenar eminence Interossei (1st most obvious)	–
	Posture	–	Partial claw hand	Wrist drop
	Sensory	Pain / sensory loss as above	Pain / sensory loss as above	Pain / sensory loss as above
	Motor	Weak thumb ABduction	Weak finger ABduction	Weak finger / wrist extension
	Tests	Tinel / Phalen +ve	Froment's sign	–

Note that a C7 radiculopathy causes a similar motor deficit to radial nerve palsy, but with sensory loss in the index and middle fingers rather than on the dorsal 1st interosseous space [see diagram on p32]

T_1 lesion
• Aetiology
  ○ Cervical spondylosis
  ○ Pancoast tumour
  ○ Plexus trauma / birth injury (Klumpke's palsy)
• Clinical features
  ○ Total claw hand (all lumbricals lost)
  ○ Wasting of small muscles in hand
  ○ Pain / sensory loss in medial forearm
  ○ Horner's syndrome may co-exist

ΔΔ Carpal tunnel syndrome
• Idiopathic (majority of case)
• Pregnancy
• RA
• Hypothyroid
• Diabetes
• Acromegaly

* Saturday night palsy = compression of the radial nerve against the humerus by falling asleep with your arm over the back of a chair

NOTES

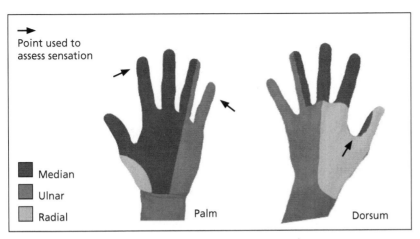

→ Point used to assess sensation

■ Median
■ Ulnar
■ Radial

Palm   Dorsum

Fig. 1. Sensory innervation of the left hand by the peripheral nerves

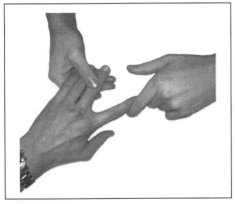

Fig. 2. Assessment of finger ABduction (Ulnar nerve)

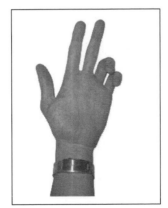

Fig. 3. Partial claw hand (Ulnar palsy)

Patient is asked to hold piece of paper between index finger and a *straight* thumb

Paper is then pulled away from patient:

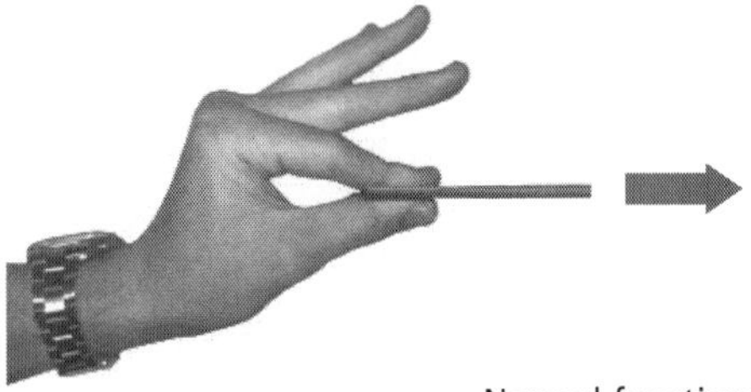

Normal function
(Thumb DIP joint remains extended)

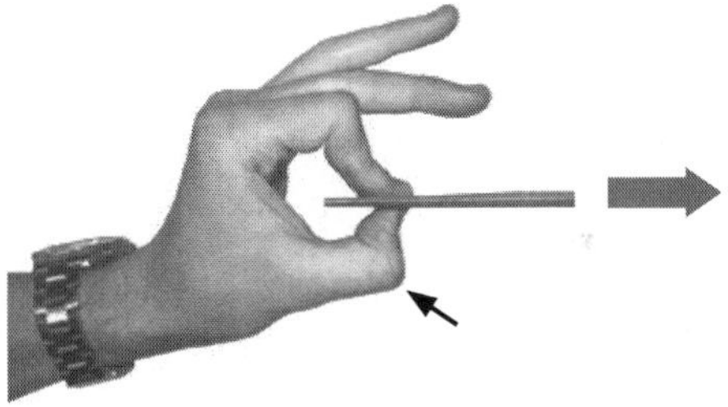

Froment's sign
(Thumb DIP joint flexes as long flexors compensate for ADductor pollicis weakness)

Fig. 4. Froment's sign (ulnar palsy)

	Action / Examine for	ΔΔ / Potential findings / Extra information
Introduction	<ul><li>Wash hands</li><li>Introduce yourself, explain examination & gain consent</li><li>Position (ideally supine at 45° but most of examination can be done seated)</li></ul>	
General inspection	<ul><li>Poverty of facial expression<ul><li>'Mask-like' face</li><li>Loss of facial micro-movements</li></ul></li><li>Flexed extrapyramidal posture<ul><li>Cannot lie flat (head held off pillow)</li><li>'Simian posture' on standing<ul><li>stooped</li><li>hands held in front of groins</li></ul></li></ul></li></ul>	→ 'Hands over hernias' position

Core features of parkinsonism (TRAP)

	Action / Examine for	ΔΔ / Potential findings / Extra information
Tremor	<ul><li>Look for Parkinsonian tremor with hands resting on a pillow<ul><li>Coarse tremor (3–4 Hz)</li><li>Pill-rolling quality</li></ul></li><li>Ask pt to hold hands out in front of them, fingers spread<ul><li>Parkinsonian tremor should improve</li></ul></li><li>Consider other causes of tremor<ul><li>Tremor which worsens with hands held up</li><li>Titubation (no–no or yes–yes head movement)</li><li>Flapping tremor – assess formally if you suspect this</li></ul></li></ul>	 → Hallmark of true resting tremor → Postural tremor → Essential tremor [⇨] → Hepatic / respiratory / renal failure
Rigidity	<ul><li>"Let your arm go completely floppy"</li><li>Take hand in 'shaking hands' grip, supporting arm at elbow</li><li>Pronate / supinate to detect supinator catch</li><li>Flex / extend wrist</li><li>Flex / extend elbow</li><li>"Tap your knee with your other hand" – continue to flex / extend elbow</li><li>Repeat with other arm</li></ul>	 → 'Cogwheeling' in parkinsonism → Synkinesis – reinforces hypertonia
Akinesia	<ul><li>Ask pt to touch thumb to each finger in turn, as quickly as possible</li><li>Hold hands out in front & pretend to play piano</li></ul>	→ 'Bradykinesia' is a more accurate description → Look for slowness in these movements

Postural instability	• Ask pt to rise from chair, walk across room, turn & come back
	• Look for parkinsonian features
	  ○ Hesitancy
	  ○ Shuffling gait
	  ○ Loss of arm swing
	  ○ Hurried steps
	  ○ Festination
	  ○ Retropulsion
		→ Slow to rise from chair, move off & turn around
		→ The 'marche à petit pas'
		
		→ Speeding up inadvertently
		→ Falling backwards as feet rush ahead

Other tests	• Glabellar tap
	  ○ Ask pt to fix eyes on a point on the wall
	  ○ "*I am going to tap on your forehead*"
	  ○ Tap repeatedly between their eyes with your index finger
	  ○ Look for failure of attenuation of the blink response
	• Speech
	  ○ Ask pt to state name & date of birth
	  ○ Listen for slow, monotonous speech
	• Writing
	  ○ Ask pt to write name & address
	  ○ Look for micrographia
	  ○ May also highlight functional difficulty
		→ In the normal individual blinking will stop after 2–3 taps
		
		→ Small handwriting

Function	• Ask pt to make motion of turning a tap • Undo then do up a button • Handle some coins	

Concluding remarks	• Assess for evidence of a Parkinson-plus syndrome
	  ○ Full neurological examination
	  ○ Erect & supine BP
	  ○ Eye movements
		→ Multi-system atrophy
		→ Shy–Drager syndrome
		→ Progressive supranuclear palsy

Core features of parkinsonism (TRAP) – Use this to guide examination sequence
- **T**remor
- **R**igidity
- **A**kinesia (or more accurately bradykinesia)
- **P**ostural instability

Causes of parkinsonism
- Idiopathic Parkinson's disease
- Drug-induced parkinsonism
  - Lithium
  - Phenothiazine antipsychotics
  - Atypical antipsychotics (less so)
  - Metoclopramide
- Parkinson-plus syndrome
  - Shy–Drager syndrome (autonomic failure)
  - Multi-system atrophy (cerebellar and pyramidal features)
  - Progressive supranuclear palsy (ocular features, including failure of vertical gaze)
- Atherosclerotic pseudoparkinsonism (legs only, less tremor)
- Dementia pugilistica
  - Parkinsonism secondary to repeated head trauma associated with boxing (e.g. Mohammed Ali)

Conditions with similar presentations to parkinsonism
- Benign essential tremor
- Wilson's disease
  - Tremor
  - Dyskinesias
  - Psychiatric illness
  - Hepatotoxicity
  - Kayser–Fleischer rings in eyes

Treatments used in Parkinson's disease
- L-dopa
- Dopamine agonists
  - Ropinerole
  - Apomorphine SC infusion
  - (Bromocriptine – disused due to SEs)
- Anticholinergics
  - Procyclidine
  - Orphenadrine
- COMT inhibitors
  - Entacapone
- MAO-B inhibitors
  - Selegiline
- Glutamate antagonists
  - Amantadine

Long-term complications of L-dopa therapy
- Increasingly severe parkinsonism
- Autonomic neuropathy
- Dysphagia
- Dementia
- Dyskinesias
- Motor fluctuations (on–off / end of dose)

NOTES

Tremor Notes

You may be asked to examine purely tremor rather than the entire extrapyramidal system. Remember that often tremors do not conform to textbook descriptions.

ΔΔ Tremor
- Resting: Parkinsonism
- Flapping: Hepatic failure (encephalopathy), respiratory failure (CO_2 retention), renal failure
- Intention: Cerebellar lesion
- Postural: Benign essential tremor, physiological tremor [see below]

	Benign essential tremor	Exaggerated physiological tremor
Aetiology	• Unknown • Genetic component likely (family history in 50%)	• Fever • Hyperthyroidism • Anxiety states • Medication-induced (e.g. β_2-agonists)
Other information	• Improvement with alcohol • Progressive	• Non-progressive
Examination	• Mild asymmetry common • Slower (~7 Hz) • Titubation in 50% • Postural & action	• Usually symmetrical • Faster (~5 Hz) • No titubation • Usually purely postural (abolished on action)
Management	• β-blockers • Gabapentin if contraindicated	• Treat / remove cause if possible • β-blockers (or gabapentin) sometimes needed

12. CEREBELLAR FUNCTION

	Action / Examine for	ΔΔ / Potential findings / Extra information
Introduction	• Wash hands • Introduce yourself, explain examination & gain consent • Expose & position pt (ideally down to shorts/pants, supine at 45°)	→ Always consider pt's dignity
General inspection	• Bruising, scars • Symmetry, muscle wasting, fasciculation	→ Recurrent falls → LMN lesion [p32]

Head		
Nystagmus	• *"Keep your head still and follow my finger"* • Move finger up, down, left & right quickly to elicit nystagmus	→ Nystagmus may be cerebellar [⇨]
Speech	• Ask pt to read something aloud • Ask pt to say 'baby hippopotamus'	→ Staccato speech → Slurring

Upper limbs		
Tone	• Assess as per upper limb neurological exam [p30]	→ Hypotonia
Power	• Assess as per upper limb neurological exam [p30]	→ Reduced power may cause apparent impairment of co-ordination even in the absence of a cerebellar lesion

Co-ordination	• Rebound test
	  ○ Ask pt to put arms out straight in front, palms down and close eyes
	  ○ *"Keep your arms in that position"*
	  ○ Push each arm down in turn ~10 cm then release it
	  ○ Watch for arm bouncing back up to beyond original position
	• Finger–nose test
	  ○ Ask pt to touch their nose with one index finger
	  ○ Place your index finger directly in front of them ~50 cm away
	  ○ Ask to cycle between nose and your finger
	  ○ Slowly move your finger away from the pt so that they must stretch arm fully to touch it
	• Hand slapping test
	  ○ Ask if left- or right-handed then demonstrate test
	  ○ For example, left hand out, palm up
	  ○ Rest right hand in left hand, palm up
	  ○ Turn right hand over in left hand, to palm down
	  ○ Alternate right hand between palm up and down
	  ○ Look for slowness and difficulty
		→ Overshoot = dysmetria
		
		→ Dysmetria, past-pointing
		→ Intention tremor (more likely to be seen at extent of arm stretch)
		
		→ Always more difficult on non-dominant side
		
		→ Dysdiadochokinesis

Lower limbs		
Tone	• Assess as per lower limb neurological exam [p34]	→ Hypotonia
Power	• Assess as per lower limb neurological exam [p34]	→ As above

Co-ordination	• Foot tapping
	  ○ Ask pt to tap foot on floor as rapidly as possible
	  ○ Look for slowness and difficulty
	• Heel–shin test
	  ○ At first guide pt through sequence by moving foot for them
	  ○ Heel onto knee
	  ○ Slide heel down front of shin
	  ○ Lift off, bring foot back up and onto knee
		→ Dysdiadochokinesis
		
		→ Intention tremor, dysmetria

Posture / gait		

Posture	• *"How stable are you when sitting or standing up?"*
	• Assess stability sitting
	  ○ Sit on side of bed
	  ○ Ask to cross arms in front and sit still
	• Assess stability standing (only if stable sitting)
	  ○ Feet together, arms by sides
	• Romberg's test
	  ○ Stand pt up, feet together, facing you
	  ○ Hover your hands above pt's shoulders
	  ○ *"Now close your eyes. I will catch you if necessary."*
	  ○ If pt suddenly becomes very unsteady – positive test
	  ○ Steady pt's shoulders and instruct to open eyes
		→ Truncal ataxia
		
		→ Truncal ataxia
		
		→ Sensory ataxia (i.e. non-cerebellar)
		
		→ Without visual input and with impaired proprioception pt cannot maintain balance

Gait	• Ask pt to walk across room and back, look for features of cerebellar gait
	  ○ Wide-based gait
	  ○ Unsteadiness with lateral veering
	  ○ Irregular steps
	• Ask to walk heel–toe
		→ Very difficult if cerebellar lesion

| Concluding remarks | • *"I would like to complete a full neurological examination"*
• Investigations: MRI for visualising posterior fossa | |

Causes of cerebellar disease
- Stroke
- Tumour
- MS
- Congenital (e.g. Arnold–Chiari)
- Friedreich's ataxia
- Alcohol abuse
- Thiamine deficiency (e.g. Wernicke's encephalopathy)
- Anti-epileptic medication

Localising the cerebellar lesion
- This may be impossible clinically
- Lesions may involve both the vermis and hemispheres
- Central (vermis) lesion symptoms tend to cause:
  - Truncal ataxia sitting & standing
  - Poor heel–toe
  - Slurred staccato speech
- Cerebellar hemisphere lesion symptoms tend to cause:
  - *Ipsilateral* limb ataxia (dysmetria, intention tremor, dysdiadochokinesis)
  - Nystagmus
  - Unsteady gait, falling towards side of lesion when walking

Classic signs of cerebellar lesion (DANISH)
- **D**ysdiadochokinesis
- **A**taxia (limb / trunk)
- **N**ystagmus
- **I**ntention tremor
- **S**peech (slurred, staccato)
- **H**ypotonia

Features of cerebellar limb ataxia
- Dysmetria
- Past-pointing
- Intention tremor
- Dysdiadochokinesis

ΔΔ Nystagmus
- Congenital (tends to cause pendular nystagmus most marked in neutral position)
- Brainstem problem (e.g. INO)
  - MS
  - Stroke
  - Tumour
- Cerebellar problem
  - See list above
  - Particularly MS
- Vestibular apparatus problem (nystagmus tends to be worse when looking away from side of lesion)
  - Labyrinthitis
  - Ménière's disease
  - CN VIII lesion

NOTES

ΔΔ Dysarthria

- Facial nerve palsy (CN VII) – look for facial weakness
- Bulbar palsy – look for flaccid, wasted, fasciculating tongue
  - MND
  - Guillain–Barré
  - Syringobulbia
- Pseudobulbar palsy – look for spastic, contracted tongue
  - MND
  - MS
  - Bilateral stroke (e.g. internal capsule)
- Myasthenia gravis
- Cerebellar disease [see above]

Wernicke's encephalopathy

- Syndrome resulting from thiamine (vitamin B_1) deficiency
- Most cases result from alcohol abuse
- If untreated (with IV thiamine replacement) may progress to irreversible Korsakoff's psychosis
- Classical clinical triad
  1. Acute confusional state
  2. Ophthalmoplegia (especially upgaze)
  3. Ataxia (and other cerebellar signs)

NOTES

Examination for signs of Cushing's syndrome

	Action / Examine for	ΔΔ / Potential findings / Extra information
Introduction	• Wash hands • Introduce yourself, explain examination & gain consent • Expose & position pt (top off, supine at 45°)	
General inspection	• Central obesity • Peripheral muscle wasting	→ This combination results in the classical 'orange on matchsticks' appearance of Cushing's
Hands	• Reduced skin fold thickness	→ Skin may feel like tissue paper
Arms	• Bruising • *"I would like to measure blood pressure"*	→ Fragile blood vessels → Hypertension
Face	• Moon facies • Acne • Plethora • Hirsutism	
Chest / back	• Gynaecomastia in male • Interscapular fat pad – 'buffalo hump' • Supraclavicular fat pads • Kyphosis	→ Vertebral wedge # due to osteoporosis
Abdomen	• Purple striae • Central obesity	
Proximal myopathy	• Test shoulder ABduction power • Ask pt to stand from chair with arms crossed (hip girdle strength)	
Legs	• Bruising	

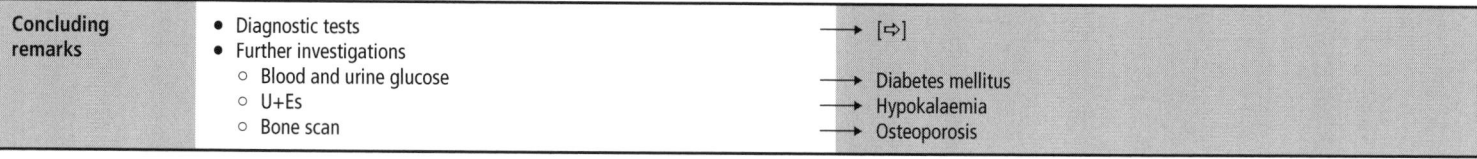

	Action / Examine for	ΔΔ / Potential findings / Extra information

Concluding remarks	• Diagnostic tests
	• Further investigations
	   ○ Blood and urine glucose
	   ○ U+Es
	   ○ Bone scan
		→ [⇨]
		
		→ Diabetes mellitus
		→ Hypokalaemia
		→ Osteoporosis

13. ENDOCRINE

Examination for signs of acromegaly

	Action / Examine for	ΔΔ / Potential findings / Extra information
Introduction	• Wash hands • Introduce yourself, explain examination & gain consent • Position pt (supine at 45° or sitting)	
General inspection	• Height • General size	→ Pt with acromegaly may be very tall or may be of normal height with large features

Hands	• Size
	• Pinch skin to assess skin fold thickness
	• Median nerve exam
	  ○ Thenar eminence wasting
	  ○ Thumb ABduction
	  ○ Sensation in lateral index finger
	  ○ Tinel / Phalen tests
	• Feel palms
		→ May be very large
		→ May be increased
		→ Carpal tunnel syndrome [p38]
		
		→ Boggy, sweaty palms indicate active disease

Arms	• "I would now measure blood pressure"	→ Hypertension
Neck	• JVP • Goitre	→ May be raised in cardiomyopathy → Due to ↑growth hormone (note pt will be euthyroid)

Face	• Prominent supraorbital ridges
	• Prognathism (best seen from side)
	• Big ears, nose and lips
	• Large tongue
	• "Show me your gums"
	  ○ Prognathism causing underbite
	  ○ Wide separation of teeth
		
		→ Enlarged, protruding mandible
		
		→ ΔΔ Amyloidosis

Eyes	• Visual fields	→ Bitemporal hemianopia (often remains after surgery)
Proximal myopathy	• Test shoulder ABduction power • Ask pt to stand from chair with arms crossed (hip girdle strength)	

Concluding remarks	• "I would arrange an oral glucose tolerance test with growth hormone and IGF-1 measurement"
	• Perform full cardiovascular examination
	• Further investigations
	  ○ Blood and urine glucose
	  ○ MRI
	  ○ ECG
		→ Failure of GH suppression confirms diagnosis
		
		→ Hypertension & cardiomyopathy
		
		→ Diabetes mellitus
		→ Pituitary adenoma
		→ Cardiomyopathy

Cushing's syndrome
- Cardiovascular system
  - Hypertension
  - Fluid retention & overload
- Gastrointestinal system
  - Fatty liver
  - Pancreatitis
- Neurological system
  - Euphoria
  - Depression
  - Psychosis
  - Insomnia
- Locomotor system
  - Proximal myopathy
  - Osteoporosis
  - Vertebral wedge fractures
  - Avascular necrosis (e.g. femoral head)
- Immune system
  - Immunosuppression
- Endocrine system
  - Diabetes mellitus
- General cushingoid features
  - Central obesity
  - Muscle wasting in limbs
  - Thin skin
  - Bruising
  - Moon facies
  - Facial plethora
  - Acne
  - Hirsutism
  - Buffalo hump
  - Gynaecomastia
  - Purple abdominal striae

Causes of Cushing's syndrome
- High ACTH
  - Pituitary adenoma (Cushing's disease)
  - Ectopic ACTH (e.g. SCLC)
- Low ACTH
  - Adenoma of adrenal cortex
  - Carcinoma of adrenal cortex
  - Iatrogenic (corticosteroid therapy)

Investigation of non-iatrogenic Cushing's syndrome
1. Preliminary diagnosis
   - Overnight dexamethasone suppression test
     or
   - 24-hour urinary free cortisol
2. Confirm diagnosis
   - 48-hour dexamethasone suppression test
3. Localise lesion
   - Plasma ACTH
   - High dose dexamethasone suppression test (some response suggests Cushing's disease)
   - Imaging: CT (chest / adrenals), MRI (pituitary fossa)

NOTES

Common indications for long-term corticosteroid Rx

- Respiratory
  - Asthma
  - COPD
  - Pulmonary fibrosis
- Gastrointestinal
  - Inflammatory bowel disease
  - Autoimmune hepatitis
- Rheumatology
  - RA
  - SLE
  - Polymyalgia rheumatica
  - GCA
  - Vasculitis
  - Myositis
- Dermatology
  - Psoriasis
  - Severe eczema
  - Pemphigus & pemphigoid
- Transplant
- Replacement doses (should not cause Cushing's)
  - Addison's disease
  - Hypopituitarism

Treatment of acromegaly

- Trans-sphenoidal resection of tumour
- Bromocriptine / octreotide
  - Reduce growth hormone synthesis
  - Used in young adults due to high risk of infertility following surgery
  - May be used pre-operatively

ΔΔ Proximal myopathy

- Cushing's syndrome
- Acromegaly
- Hyperthyroidism
- Muscular dystrophy
- Polymyositis
- Dermatomyositis
- Myasthenia gravis
- Hypo / hyper K^+
- Hypo / hyper Ca^{2+}

Features of dermatomyositis

- Proximal myopathy
- Heliotrope facial rash
- Gottron's papules (extensor surfaces of fingers)

NOTES

	Action / Examine for	ΔΔ / Potential findings / Extra information
Introduction	• Wash hands • Introduce yourself, explain examination & gain consent • Expose pt (xiphisternum to pubic symphysis) • Position pt (semi-recumbent) • *"Do you have any pain in your tummy?"* • *"How many weeks pregnant are you?"*	→ Lying flat can obstruct IVC & cause symptomatic hypotension

The abdomen

	Action / Examine for	ΔΔ / Potential findings / Extra information

Inspection	• Abdominal distension
	• Fetal movements
	• Scars
	  ○ Pfannenstiel (transverse suprapubic)
	  ○ Laparotomy
	  ○ Laparoscopic
	• Cutaneous signs of pregnancy
	  ○ Linea nigra
	  ○ Striae gravidarum
	  ○ Striae albicans
	  ○ Umbilical inversion
	  ○ Dilated superficial veins
		→ The 6 Fs: Fat, Fluid, Flatus, Faeces, Fetus, Flipping big mass
		→ Present from 24 wks
		
		→ Caesarian section
		→ Ruptured ectopic, ovarian mass removal
		→ Various gynaecological procedures
		
		→ Dark line down central abdomen from xiphisternum to pubis
		→ Purple straie (no clinical significance)
		→ Silvery-white striae (previous parity)
		→ Increased intra-abdominal pressure
		→ Collateral flow due to pressure on IVC from gravid uterus

Palpation	• Fundal height
	  ○ *"I'm going to feel for the top of your womb"*
	  ○ Use left hand, start at xiphisternum
	  ○ Work down until fundus located
	  ○ Place end of tape measure here
	  ○ Measure to pubic symphysis *with measurements facing downwards*
	  ○ Pinch tape measure at pubic symphysis & turn over to obtain measurement
	• Fetal lie (and number of fetuses)
	  ○ *"I'm now going to feel for your baby"*
	  ○ Watch pt's face throughout
	  ○ One hand each side of uterus
	  ○ Apply gentle pressure with left hand
	  ○ With right hand feel for firm, curved fetal back or lumpy fetal limbs
	  ○ Apply pressure with right hand & feel with left as above
		
		→ Uterus palpable from 12 wks, reaches umbilicus at 20 wks
		
		→ Avoids bias
		→ Fundal height in cm +/− 3 = weeks' gestation (after 20 wks)
		
		→ Relationship of longitudinal axes of fetus and uterus
		
		→ To ensure you do not cause any pain
		
		→ Stabilises fetus
		
		→ Lie can be longitudinal, oblique or transverse

	• Presenting part	→ Part of fetus overlying pelvic brim
	○ *"I'm going to feel deeply for the baby; if this is painful please tell me"*	
	○ Continue to watch pt's face	
	○ One hand each side of lower uterus, just above pubic symphysis	
	○ Apply firm pressure with both hands	
	○ Decide if hard, narrow & round (head) or soft and broad (bottom)	
	• Engagement of the head	→ Cephalic = presenting head, breech = presenting bottom
	○ Determine cephalic presentation (as above)	→ 'Engaged' = widest part of fetal head has entered pelvis
	○ Approximate how many finger breadths are needed to cover head above pelvic brim	
	○ Describe as 'fifths (of head) palpable'	→ One finger breadth = 1/5; ≤3/5 palpable = engaged
Auscultation	• Consider fetal lie & palpate anterior shoulder	
	• Pinard stethoscope	→ Can be used after 24 wks' gestation
	○ Place bell over anterior shoulder	
	○ Press firmly but gently into abdomen	
	○ Put ear to other end	→ Auscultate for 1 min (normal 120–140 bpm)
	• Doppler ultrasound	→ Can be used after 18 wks' gestation
	○ Smear jelly on probe	
	○ Place probe over anterior shoulder	
	○ Adjust angle until clear heartbeat heard	→ Listen for 1 min (normal 120–140 bpm)
Legs	• Peripheral oedema	→ Can be physiological or occur with pre-eclampsia [⇨]
Concluding remarks	• Cardio-respiratory examination	
	• Blood pressure	→ Pre-existing HTN, gestational HTN, pre-eclampsia
	• Urinalysis	→ Proteinuria (e.g. pre-eclampsia), glycosuria (gestational DM)
	• USS	
	• Cardiotocography if abnormal heart rate	

Pre-eclampsia = Pregnancy-induced hypertension + proteinuria (>0.3 g in 24 hours) +/– oedema

ΔΔ Large fundal height
- Macrosomia
- Multiple pregnancy
- Polyhydramnios

Intrauterine growth restriction
- Maternal causes
  - Increasing maternal age
  - Smoking
  - Alcohol
  - Infections (CMV, toxo, rubella, syphilis)
  - Diabetes mellitus (including gestational)
  - Renal disease
  - Hypertension
  - Thrombophilia
  - Drugs (warfarin, phenytoin, steroids)
- Placental causes
  - Pre-eclampsia
  - Placental abruption
- Fetal causes
  - Chromosomal abnormalities
  - Anencephaly
  - Multiple pregnancy

ΔΔ Small fundal height
- Fetal descent into pelvis before delivery
- Intrauterine growth retardation
- Oligohydramnios

Risk factors for breech presentation
- High maternal parity (lax uterus)
- Uterine anomaly
- Placenta praevia
- Pelvic bony abnormality
- Smoking
- Diabetes
- Fetal malformation (e.g. hydrocephalus)
- Multiple pregnancy
- Poly- or oligohydramnios
- Low birth weight (preterm delivery or IUGR)
- Previous breech delivery

PREGNANT ABDOMEN NOTES

Physiological changes in pregnancy

- Cardiovascular
  - Cardiac output increases 30–50% (both heart rate and stroke volume increase)
  - Reduced systemic vascular resistance due to progesterone and response to placental invasion (may cause postural hypotension)
  - BP falls during mid-pregnancy and returns to normal by week 36
  - Impaired venous return from the IVC due to pressure from the gravid uterus in late pregnancy
  - RAAS activation, salt & water retention, peripheral oedema
- Respiratory
  - Increased tidal volume
  - Compensated respiratory alkalosis (lower maternal pCO_2 facilitates placental gas transfer)
- Gastrointestinal
  - Increased appetite
  - Lower oesophageal sphincter relaxation due to progesterone (predisposes to reflux symptoms)
  - Reduced GI tract motility & increased transit time (constipation common)
  - Gallbladder dilatation & incomplete emptying (predisposes to gallstone formation)
- Urinary
  - Increased renal blood flow & GFR
  - Ureteric & bladder relaxation due to progesterone (increases risk of UTI)
- Endocrine
  - Increasing progesterone & oestrogen
  - Suppressed FSH & LH
  - Increased ACTH and cortisol
  - Increased prolactin
  - Increased T4/T3 but also increased thyroxine-binding globulin
  - Reduced peripheral insulin sensitivity (predisposes to gestational diabetes)
- Haematological
  - Increased plasma volume & dilutional anaemia
  - Slightly raised white cell count
  - Reduced serum iron, increased transferrin & TIBC
  - Increased clotting factors (VII, VIII, IX, X) and reduced fibrinolytic activity (predisposes to VTE)
- Skin
  - Hyperpigmentation of umbilicus, nipples, abdominal midline (linea nigra) and face (chloasma)
  - Striae gravidarum
  - Palmar erythema (hyperdynamic circulation)
- Musculoskeletal
  - Increased ligament laxity (causes back pain & pubic symphysis dysfunction)
  - Exaggerated lumbar lordosis in late pregnancy

SURGERY

Action / Examine for	ΔΔ / Potential findings / Extra information
Introduction	<ul><li>Wash hands</li><li>Introduce yourself, explain examination & gain consent</li><li>Expose & position pt (sleeves rolled past elbows, hands on a pillow)</li><li>*"Do you have any pain in the joints of your hands or arms?"*</li></ul>	

Musculoskeletal assessment

Look	

- Palms facing down (look step-wise from wrists to nails)
  - Wrists
    - swelling   → RA
    - radiocarpal subluxation   → RA
    - prominent ulnar styloid   → RA
  - Dorsum
    - tight, cold, waxy skin with telangectasia   → Scleroderma
    - muscle wasting   → RA, nerve palsy [p40]
    - rheumatoid nodules   → Seropositive RA
  - MCP joints
    - swelling   → RA
    - ulnar deviation   → RA
    - subluxation / dislocation   → RA
  - Fingers
    - scars   → Previous surgery for RA / OA / #
    - swelling   → RA
    - swan-neck, boutonniere, Z-thumb   → RA (Z-thumb = boutonniere of thumb)
    - spindling   → RA, scleroderma
    - Heberden's (DIP) & Bouchard's (PIP) nodes   → OA – remember 'Outer *Heber*dies'
  - Nails
    - pitting, onycholysis   → Psoriasis
    - nailfold infarcts   → Vasculitis, SLE
    - clubbing, leuconychia, koilonychia   → Remote pathology [p112]
- Palms facing upwards
  - Palmar erythema   → RA, CLD, hyperthyroidism, pregnancy
- Praying position
  - Palms together, bring elbows up so wrist extended to ~90°
  - Look for fixed flexion deformity of fingers   → RA, scleroderma, Dupuytren's, OA
- Make fists
  - Loss of 'valleys' between metacarpal heads   → RA (MCP swelling)
  - Limitation of finger flexion
  - Ask to straighten fingers quickly – look for finger 'triggering'   → Tenosynovitis (idiopathic), RA
- Fists up to chin exposing forearms and elbows
  - Rheumatoid nodules   → Seropositive RA
  - Psoriasis   → Possible psoriatic arthropathy
- Ears, neck & scalp
  - Psoriasis   → Possible psoriatic arthropathy
  - Gouty tophi on ears   → Chronic tophaceous gout

Feel
(and passive movement)
	• Feel palm for Dupuytren's contracture
	• Palpate any nodes or nodules
	• Temperature – use back of your hand and compare sides
	   ○ Dorsal wrist & MCP joints
	• Squeeze across each joint then passively flex & extend
	   ○ Wrists
	   ○ MCP joints (if any pain assess individual joints more carefully)
	   ○ Small joints of fingers & thumbs
		→ CLD, diabetes, heavy labour, phenytoin, trauma, familial
		
		→ Active RA
		   ○ Hot, red, swollen joints
		   ○ Tender on palpation
		   ○ Painful passive flexion

Move 1: **Hand function**	• Squeeze: Ask pt to squeeze your index and middle finger tightly • Pinch: Ask pt to touch thumb to each of their fingers in turn • Piano: Ask pt to hold hands out and wiggle fingers • Button: Ask pt to undo then do up a button	→ Power grip → Precision grip → Crude assessment of hand function → Assesses precision hand function

Move 2:
Upper limb
function
	• Ask pt to complete this sequence of movements
	   ○ Put arms straight out (elbow extension)
	   ○ Cock wrists back (wrist extension)
	   ○ 'Turn the taps on and off' (pronation / supination)
	   ○ Bring hands into chest (elbow flexion)
	   ○ Put hands behind head (shoulder ABduction & ext rotation)
	   ○ Slide hands up back (shoulder internal rotation)
		→ Important to quickly assess entire upper limb function (should take less than 30 sec)
		
		→ Able to dress
		→ Able to clean after toilet

Neurological assessment (optional depending on context of case, but usually worth doing quickly)		
Sensation	• Median: Lateral aspect of index finger • Ulnar: Medial aspect of little finger • Radial: Dorsal 1st interosseous space	→ [p41 – Fig. 1]
Power	• Median: Thumb ABduction • Ulnar: Index finger ABduction • Radial: Finger extension	→ [p38]
Special tests	• Tinel / Phalen / Froment's if indicated	→ [p38]

Concluding **remarks**	• "I would like to examine the rest of the musculoskeletal system" • Examination of other systems where applicable • Investigations: X-ray, ESR / CRP, rheumatoid factor, joint aspiration	→ Pattern of joint involvement can aid diagnosis

How to present your findings	NOTES

In the common case of a pt with barn-door features of RA
- *"There is a symmetrical, deforming polyarthropathy affecting the small joints of the hands in a rheumatoid pattern. The most common differentials for this clinical picture are RA and psoriatic arthropathy."*

'Examine this pt's hands' cases – modify your examination based on what you find
- Musculoskeletal: OA, RA, psoriatic arthropathy, gout
- Neurological: Median nerve palsy (carpal tunnel), ulnar nerve palsy (check for elbow trauma), radial nerve palsy, T1 lesion, MND
- Endocrine: Thyroid disease, acromegaly
- Remote pathology: Clubbing, leuconychia, koilonychia

RA statistics
- 3 females : 1 male
- Peak prevalence age 30–50
- 70% seropositive (as is 5% of general population)
  - Rheumatoid factor +ve (IgM against self-IgG)
  - Often have nodules
  - Extra-articular features
  - Progressive disease
- 20% of all RA pts have nodules
- 50% HLA-DR4 +ve (severe, erosive disease)

Features of *active* RA
- Inflamed joints
  - Red
  - Hot
  - Swollen
  - Tender
- Pain on passive movement
- Increased duration of morning stiffness
- Raised ESR
- Anaemia [see below]

Extra-articular features of RA
- General: Malaise, lethargy, low grade fever, weight loss
- CVS: Pericarditis, pericardial effusion
- RS: Nodules, pleural effusion, pulmonary fibrosis, pneumoconiosis (Caplan's syndrome)
- GUS: Renal amyloid
- NS: Polyneuropathy, mononeuritis multiplex, carpal tunnel, atlanto-axial subluxation
- Eyes: Scleritis, episcleritis, keratoconjunctivitis sicca, Sjögren's syndrome
- Blood: Anaemia [see below], thrombocytosis, ↓WCC (Felty's syndrome = ↓WCC + splenomegaly + RA)

Multifactorial aetiology of anaemia in RA
- Anaemia of chronic disease
- Iron deficiency anaemia secondary to NSAID-induced gastritis / peptic ulcer
- Aplastic anaemia secondary to DMARD therapy
- Macrocytic anaemia secondary to methotrexate (folate metabolism)
- Pernicious anaemia (associated with RA)

RA X-ray
- Loss of joint space
- Bony erosions
- Periarticular osteoporosis
- Deformity (e.g. subluxation)
- Soft tissue swelling

OA X-ray
- Loss of joint space
- Osteophytes
- Subchondral sclerosis
- Bone cysts

Psoriatic arthropathy
- Affects 10% of pts with psoriasis
- In 75% skin features present before arthropathy
- In 20% skin features present after arthropathy
- In 5% no skin features will ever appear

Presentations of psoriatic arthropathy
- Asymmetrical oligoarthritis
  - Mainly hands and feet (dactylitis)
  - Sometimes larger joints
- Lone DIP disease
- Rheumatoid pattern
- Arthritis mutilans
- Sacroiliitis

Sjögren's syndrome
- Dry eyes (keratoconjunctivitis sicca), dry mouth (xerostomia) & parotid gland enlargement
- May occur independently, or associated with RA / SLE / scleroderma

DMARDs & key side effects
- All DMARDS
  - Marrow suppression
  - Hepatotoxicity
  - Rash
  - GI upset (especially nausea & oral ulcers)
- Methotrexate
  - Pneumonitis & pulmonary fibrosis [p13]
  - Megalobastic anaemia
- Hydroxychloroquine
  - Retinopathy
- Sulfasalazine
  - Oligospermia
- IM Gold
  - Nephrotic syndrome
- Penicillamine
  - Nephrotic syndrome
  - Altered taste
  - Myasthenia gravis-like syndrome
- Ciclosporin
  - Renal impairment
  - HTN
  - Gum hypertrophy
- Leflunomide
- Azathioprine

	Action / Examine for	ΔΔ / Potential findings / Extra information
Introduction	• Wash hands • Introduce yourself, explain examination & gain consent • Expose & position pt (top off, standing) • *"I would like to compare the affected shoulder with the unaffected one"* • *"Which shoulder is sore? Can you point to where it is painful?"*	→ Examiner may ask you to proceed with examination of just one shoulder

Look	• From front, sides & back
	  ○ Symmetry (compare sides)
	  ○ Muscle wasting
	  ○ Scars
	  ○ Redness / swelling
	  ○ Deformity including winged scapula
	• Check axillae for obvious abnormality
		
		→ Deltoid – axillary nerve palsy
		→ Arthroscopy, shoulder replacement
		→ Inflammation
		→ Long thoracic nerve palsy

Feel	• Temperature
	  ○ Use back of hand & compare sides
	  ○ Anterior & posterior shoulder
	• Bony anatomy – *"Tell me if I cause you any discomfort"*
	  ○ Palpate sternoclavicular joint, clavicle & AC joint
	  ○ Palpate anterior joint, long head of biceps & posterior joint
	  ○ Palpate borders of scapula
		→ Warmth indicates inflammation
		
		→ Feel for tenderness, bony abnormality (e.g. osteophytes)

Move 1: Formal joint assessment	• Assess ROM and pain on movement
	• Active movement
	  ○ Looking from the side
	    ■ flexion
	    ■ extension
	    ■ external rotation with elbows flexed to 90°
	  ○ Looking from behind
	    ■ ABduction
	    ■ slow ABduction as you stabilise tip of scapula
	    ■ internal rotation (reach up middle of back)
	• Passive movement – *"Tell me if I cause you any discomfort"*
	  ○ All above movements with hand on top of shoulder
	  ○ Slow ABduction to detect painful arc
		
		→ Both shoulders at once (unless you have been told to examine one only)
		→ Normal 180°
		→ Normal 60°
		→ Normal 70°
		
		→ Normal 180°
		→ Ratio of true gleno-humeral to scapular movement (normally 2:1)
		→ Each shoulder in turn
		→ Feel for crepitus
		→ Impingement syndrome [⇨]

Move 2: Functional assessment	• Both hands behind head • Both hands up to mouth • Both hands down to bottom	→ Washing hair, dressing → Eating → Cleaning after toilet

Special tests (divided by the pathology which they test for)	• Shoulder instability – shoulder apprehension test	→ Young pts, usually previous dislocation
	○ Best done with pt supine	→ All other tests conducted standing
	○ 'That's how for now' position	→ [⇨ Fig. 5]
	○ ABduct shoulder 90°, flex elbow 90°, externally rotate shoulder	→ Forearm nearing horizontal
	○ Stabilise pt's elbow with one hand	
	○ Force further external rotation with other hand	→ Push downwards on pt's hand
	○ 'Apprehensive' reaction to this = positive test	
	• Impingement syndrome – Hawkin's test	→ Middle-aged pts
	○ Flex shoulder 90°, flex elbow 90°, internally rotate shoulder	→ Forearm pointing downwards
	○ Stabilise pt's elbow with one hand	
	○ Force further internal rotation with other hand	→ Push downwards on pt's hand
	○ Pain in shoulder = positive test	
	• Rotator cuff injury (supraspinatus) – Jobe's test	→ Older pts
	○ 'Gladiator' position	
	○ Straight arm ABducted to 90°, thumb pointed at floor	
	○ "Keep your arm up, don't let me push it down"	
	○ Force shoulder ADduction against resistance from pt	→ Push downwards on pt's hand
	○ Pain / difficulty = positive test	→ May also be painful if impingement present
	• Rotator cuff injury (subscapularis) – Gerber's lift-off test	→ Older pts
	○ Hand behind back, dorsum resting against mid-lumbar spine	
	○ Stand behind pt	
	○ Apply light pressure to pt's outward-facing palm	
	○ "Push your hand straight backwards, off your back"	
	○ Pain / difficulty = positive test	
	• Rotator cuff injury (teres minor & infraspinatus) – resisted external rotation	→ Older pts
	○ Arms by sides, elbows flexed to 90°	
	○ Ask to externally rotate shoulders whilst you oppose them	→ Apply 'inwards' pressure to hands
	○ Pain / difficulty = positive test	
Neurovascular integrity	• Sensation	
	○ Axillary: Regimental badge area	→ Anterior shoulder dislocation
	○ Median: Lateral aspect of index finger	→ [p41]
	○ Ulnar: Medial aspect of little finger	
	○ Radial: Dorsal 1st interosseous space	
	• Radial pulse & CRT in finger	
Concluding remarks	• If not done: "I would like to examine the other shoulder"	
	• "I would like to examine the rest of the musculoskeletal system"	→ Pattern of joint involvement can aid diagnosis
	• Investigations: X-rays (AP & modified axillary views), MRI, joint aspiration	

Common shoulder pathology

1. Instability
- Usually young pt
- Previous dislocation(s)
- Shoulder apprehension test

2. Impingement syndrome
- Usually middle-aged pt
- Hawkin's test

3. Rotator cuff tear
- Usually older pt
- Remember 'grey hair cuff tear'
- Muscles of rotator cuff & their relevant special tests
  - supraspinatus – anterosuperior cuff – Jobe's test
  - subscapularis – anteroinferior cuff – Gerber's lift-off test
  - teres minor & infraspinatus – posterior cuff – resisted external shoulder rotation

Complications of anterior dislocation of shoulder (95% of dislocations are anterior)

- Axillary nerve damage
- Brachial plexus / other nerve damage
- Axillary artery damage
- Associated fracture (30% of cases)
  - Humeral head
  - Clavicle
  - Acromion
- Recurrent shoulder dislocation
- Anatomical lesion
  - Bankart
  - Hill–Sachs
- Rotator cuff injury

Impingement syndrome

- Also known as painful arc syndrome
- Underlying pathology is supraspinatus tendonitis
- Painful arc
  - Classical sign of supraspinatus tendonitis
  - Pain during shoulder ABduction between 60° and 120°
  - Due to 'impingement' of the underside of the acromion on the inflamed tendon
- Positive Hawkin's test
  - Arm flexed to 90°
  - Elbow flexed to 90°
  - Shoulder internally rotated, pushing supraspinatus tendon up against acromion
  - Forcing further internal rotation causes pain if tendon is inflamed
  - (Note Jobe's test for supraspinatus weakness/tear may also cause pain)

NOTES

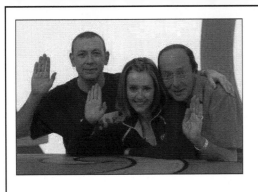

Fig. 5. Position for shoulder apprehension test (with patient supine)

The *'that's how for now'* salute was made famous by the hit children's TV show *How 2* in the 1990s. Reproduced here with permission from STV.

	Action / Examine for	ΔΔ / Potential findings / Extra information
Introduction	• Wash hands • Introduce yourself, explain examination & gain consent • Expose & position pt (down to pants or shorts, standing initially) • *"I would like to compare the affected knee with the unaffected one"* • *"Which knee is sore? Where is it sore?"*	→ Examiner may ask you to proceed with examination of just one knee

Standing & gait	• Clues to pathology (walking stick, crutch)
	• With pt standing look from front, sides & back
	  ○ Varus deformity (bow-legged)
	  ○ Valgus deformity (knock-kneed)
	• Ask pt to walk across room and back
	• Now lie pt flat with one pillow
		
		→ OA (rickets historically)
		→ Especially RA, also OA
		→ Antalgic gait (limp)

Look	• Knees
	  ○ Symmetry (compare sides)
	  ○ Muscle wasting
	  ○ Scars
	  ○ Redness
	  ○ Swelling
	  ○ Fixed flexion (look from the side)
	• Measure thigh circumference 10 cm above patella
		
		→ Arthroscopy, knee replacement
		→ Inflammation
		→ Inflammation, effusion
		→ OA, other knee pathology
		→ Hamstring / quadriceps wasting

Feel	• Temperature
	  ○ Use back of hand & compare sides
	  ○ Thigh above knee joint, medial & lateral knee
	• *"Tell me if I cause you any discomfort"*
	• With knee flexed to 90°
	  ○ Palpate medial & lateral joint lines
	  ○ Palpate patellar tendon insertion (tibial tuberosity)
	• With leg straight
	  ○ Palpate patellar border
	  ○ Palpate behind knee for swelling
	• Patellar tap
	  ○ Leg straight, compress suprapatellar bursa with one hand
	  ○ Attempt to 'bounce' patella with other hand
	• Massage test
	  ○ Leg straight, run hand up medial side of knee 2–3 times
	  ○ Immediately run hand *down* lateral side of knee
	  ○ Watch for 'bulge' of fluid in medial compartment
		→ Warmth = sign of inflammation
		
		→ Feel for tenderness, bony abnormality (e.g. osteophytes)
		
		→ Baker's cyst, popliteal aneurysm
		→ Large knee effusion
		
		→ Small knee effusion
		(more sensitive than patellar tap)

Move	• Assess ROM & pain on movement
	• Active movement
	  ○ Flexion – *"Bring your heel right into your bottom"* → Normal 140°
	  ○ Extension
	  ○ Hyperextension – *"Push the back of your knee into the bed"* → 10° hyperextension normal
	  ○ Straight leg raise – *"Keep your leg straight, raise your heel off the bed"* → Integrity of extensor mechanism
	• Passive movement – *"Tell me if this causes any discomfort"*
	  ○ Flexion & extension with hand on top of patella → Feel for crepitus

Special tests
(perform as
one sequence)
	• Anterior drawer test → ACL integrity
	  ○ Flex knee to 90°
	  ○ First look from side for posterior sag → (PCL integrity)
	  ○ Sit on pt's foot
	  ○ Grab behind knee with both hands, thumbs on tibial tuberosity
	  ○ Attempt to pull tibia forwards on the femur
	• McMurray's test → Meniscal tear
	  ○ Flex knee and hip to 90°
	  ○ Grasp sole of foot with one hand
	  ○ Grasp knee with other hand, thumb feeling down one joint line and
	    index finger feeling down the other
	  ○ Straighten knee with foot held in external then internal rotation
	  ○ Feel for 'click' and look for pt discomfort
	• Collateral ligament stress test → MCL / LCL weakness
	  ○ Flex knee to 15°
	  ○ Grasp foot with one hand, support knee with the other
	  ○ Stress each side of the knee in turn, feeling for laxity
	• Patellar apprehension test → Previous patellar dislocation
	  ○ Leg straight
	  ○ Apply lateral force to patella, begin to flex knee, watching face
	  ○ If pt 'apprehensive' and doesn't allow this = positive test

Neurovascular **integrity**	• Sensation on dorsal foot & sole of foot • Dorsalis pedis & posterior tibial pulses; CRT in hallux

Concluding **remarks**	• If not done: *"I would like to examine the other knee"* • *"I would like to examine the rest of the musculoskeletal system, in* → Pattern of joint involvement can aid diagnosis *particular the hip and ankle joints of the affected leg"* • Investigations: X-rays (2 views), MRI, aspiration of effusion

Muscles of the hamstring group (knee flexors)
- Semitendinosis
- Semimembranosus
- Biceps femoris

Knee osteoarthritis
- Very common
- May affect
  - Medial compartment
  - Lateral compartment
  - Patellofemoral compartment
  - All 3 (tricompartmental OA)
- Treatment
  - Conservative
    - analgesia
    - physiotherapy
    - walking aids
  - Operative
    - total knee replacement

Muscles of the quadriceps group (knee extensors)
- Rectus femoris
- Vastus lateralis
- Vastus intermedius
- Vastus medialis

Meniscal injuries
- Relatively common
- Young pt – likely purely traumatic tear of medial meniscus
- Older pt – increased chance of degenerative tear of lateral meniscus
- Loose meniscal fragment may enter joint space, causing locking (inability to extend knee)

Common peroneal nerve
- Anatomy
  - Descends obliquely along lateral side of popliteal fossa
  - Winds around fibular neck
  - Superficial branch innervates muscles of lateral leg compartment (foot eversion)
  - Deep branch innervates muscles of the anterior leg compartment (foot dorsiflexion)
  - Sensory supply to lateral leg and dorsum of foot
- Injury
  - Trauma to lateral leg at the level of fibular head
  - Classically being hit by a car bumper
  - Most significant consequence is loss of foot dorsiflexion, leading to foot drop
  - Results in high-stepping gait [p79]

NOTES

Acute monoarthritis / oligoarthritis

- Initial investigation
  - Make every attempt to aspirate joint & send synovial fluid for Gram stain, polarised microscopy (for crystals) & culture
  - Blood cultures
  - Inflammatory markers (FBC for WCC and differential, CRP, ESR)
  - XR
- Consider diagnosis
  - See table below for ΔΔ (**GRASP**)
  - An acutely inflamed joint is septic until proven otherwise
  - Start empirical antibiotics following joint aspiration & blood cultures if pt unwell
  - Remember haemarthrosis as a ΔΔ especially if history of clotting disorder (e.g. haemophilia)

Aetiology	Typical age	Typical gender	Typical joint involvement	Other information	Specific Ix
Gout	Middle age to elderly	Male > Female	1st MTPJ > ankle > knee > upper limb	• Polyarticular in 10%	• Serum urate
Reactive **A**rthritis	Young	Male > Female	Lower limb large joint (usually > 1 joint involved)	• Associated with GI & GUM infections • Take GI, GU & sexual history • Look for rash, balanitis, conjunctivitis	• Stool sample • STD swabs
Septic Joint	Any age	Male or Female	Any joint	• Usually staphylococcus in adults • Consider gonococcus in young adults	
Pseudogout	Middle age to elderly	Male or Female	Knee or wrist	• Can mimic gout or sepsis	• Chondrocalcinosis on XR

	Action / Examine for	ΔΔ / Potential findings / Extra information
Introduction	<ul><li>Wash hands</li><li>Introduce yourself, explain examination & gain consent</li><li>Expose & position pt (down to pants or shorts, standing initially)</li><li>*"I would like to compare the affected hip with the unaffected one"*</li><li>*"Which hip is sore? Where is it sore?"*</li></ul>	→ Examiner may ask you to proceed with examination of just one hip
Standing & gait	<ul><li>Clues to pathology (walking stick, crutch)</li><li>With pt standing look from front, sides & back</li><li>Ask pt to walk across room and back</li><li>Observe for Trendelenburg gait<ul><li>Pelvis tilts away from affected hip (as per Trendelenburg test)</li><li>Trunk tilts towards affected hip to compensate</li><li>Results in a wobbling gait</li></ul></li><li>Observe for other gait abnormalities</li><li>Now lie pt flat with one pillow</li></ul>	→ Same causes as for positive Trendelenburg test [see below] → Antalgic (limp), etc. [p79]
Look	<ul><li>Hips<ul><li>Symmetry (compare sides)</li><li>Muscle wasting</li><li>Scars</li><li>Redness</li><li>Swelling</li><li>Fixed flexion (look from the side)</li><li>External rotation of leg (look at foot)</li></ul></li><li>Measure leg length with tape measure<ul><li>True: ASIS to medial maleolus</li><li>Apparent: Umbilicus to medial maleolus</li></ul></li></ul>	 → Arthroscopy, arthroplasty, DHS → Inflammation → Inflammation, effusion → OA, other hip pathology → # NOF (acute or malunion) → [⇨] → Caused by tilting of pelvis (e.g. OA)
Feel	<ul><li>Temperature<ul><li>Use back of hand and compare sides</li><li>Anterior hip joint, over greater trochanter (lateral thigh)</li></ul></li><li>*"Tell me if I cause you any discomfort"*</li><li>Hip in neutral position<ul><li>Palpate ASIS</li><li>Palpate anterior joint line (deep)</li><li>Palpate greater trochanter (lateral)</li></ul></li></ul>	→ Warmth indicates inflammation → Feel for tenderness, bony abnormality (e.g. osteophytes) → Trochanteric bursitis (trauma, OA)

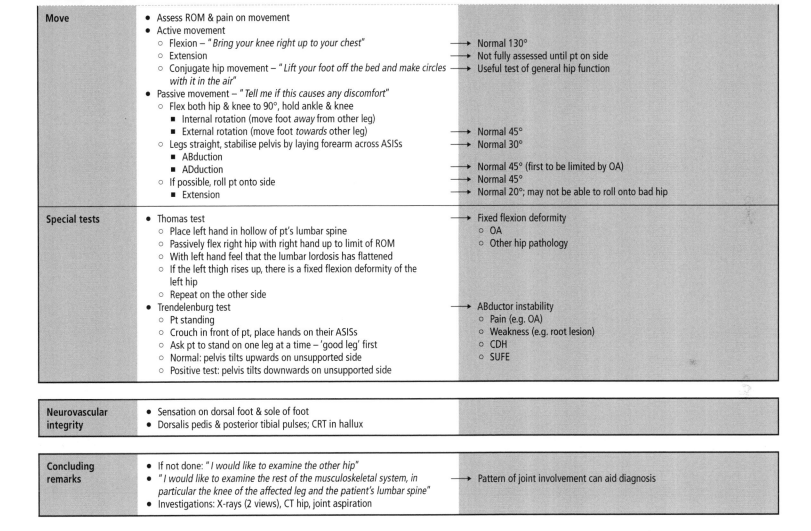

Move	• Assess ROM & pain on movement • Active movement ○ Flexion – *"Bring your knee right up to your chest"*	→ Normal 130°
	○ Extension	→ Not fully assessed until pt on side
	○ Conjugate hip movement – *"Lift your foot off the bed and make circles with it in the air"*	→ Useful test of general hip function

	• Passive movement – *"Tell me if this causes any discomfort"*
	 ○ Flex both hip & knee to 90°, hold ankle & knee
	  ▪ Internal rotation (move foot *away* from other leg)
	  ▪ External rotation (move foot *towards* other leg)
		→ Normal 45°

	○ Legs straight, stabilise pelvis by laying forearm across ASISs	→ Normal 30°
	▪ ABduction	→ Normal 45° (first to be limited by OA)
	▪ ADduction	→ Normal 45°
	○ If possible, roll pt onto side ▪ Extension	→ Normal 20°; may not be able to roll onto bad hip
Special tests	• Thomas test ○ Place left hand in hollow of pt's lumbar spine ○ Passively flex right hip with right hand up to limit of ROM ○ With left hand feel that the lumbar lordosis has flattened ○ If the left thigh rises up, there is a fixed flexion deformity of the left hip ○ Repeat on the other side	→ Fixed flexion deformity ○ OA ○ Other hip pathology
	• Trendelenburg test ○ Pt standing ○ Crouch in front of pt, place hands on their ASISs ○ Ask pt to stand on one leg at a time – 'good leg' first ○ Normal: pelvis tilts upwards on unsupported side ○ Positive test: pelvis tilts downwards on unsupported side	→ ABductor instability ○ Pain (e.g. OA) ○ Weakness (e.g. root lesion) ○ CDH ○ SUFE
Neurovascular integrity	• Sensation on dorsal foot & sole of foot • Dorsalis pedis & posterior tibial pulses; CRT in hallux	
Concluding remarks	• If not done: *"I would like to examine the other hip"* • *"I would like to examine the rest of the musculoskeletal system, in particular the knee of the affected leg and the patient's lumbar spine"* • Investigations: X-rays (2 views), CT hip, joint aspiration	→ Pattern of joint involvement can aid diagnosis

Hip flexors
- Psoas
- Iliacus
- Tensor fasciae latae
- Sartorius
- Pectineus
- ADductor longus
- ADductor brevis
- Rectus femoris (one of the quadriceps)

Leg length shortening
- Apparent – due to pelvic tilting
  - Fixed flexion deformity of hip
  - Fixed ADduction deformity of hip (especially OA)
- True – due to joint or bony abnormality
  - Pathology distal to trochanters
    - previous # femur
    - previous # tibia
    - growth disturbance (polio, epiphyseal trauma)
  - Pathology proximal to trochanters
    - # NOF
    - OA
    - hip dislocation

Hip extensors
- Gluteus maximus
- Hamstrings

Hip ABductors
- Gluteus medius & minimus

Hip ADductors
- ADductor magnus, longus & brevis

Total hip replacement
- Indications
  - OA
  - Less commonly RA / CDH / seronegative arthropathy
  - Displaced intracapsular NOF # in young pt [see below]
- Complications
  - Perioperative (anaesthetic-related, haemorrhage, infection)
  - Acute dislocation
  - Chronic infection
- Contraindications
  - Mild disease
  - Doubt as to origin of hip pain
  - Morbid obesity

NOTES

OA X-ray
- Loss of joint space
- Osteophytes
- Subchondral sclerosis
- Bone cysts

RA X-ray
- Loss of joint space
- Bony erosions
- Periarticular osteoporosis
- Deformity (e.g. subluxation)
- Soft tissue swelling

Neck of femur #
- Usually elderly, osteoporotic pt following low-velocity fall onto hip
- Blood supply to the femoral head
  1. Cervical arteries running in the joint capsule retinaculum (*main supply*)
  2. Intramedullary vessels in the femoral neck
  3. Vessels of the ligamentum teres (negligible contribution, often non-existent)
- Displaced intracapsular #
  ○ Inevitable interruption of intramedullary vessels and likely disruption of cervical arteries
  ○ High risk of avascular necrosis (AVN) of femoral head
  ○ Usually treated by hip replacement
    ▪ hemi-arthroplasty in older pts
    ▪ total hip replacement in younger pts likely to be more active post-op
- Undisplaced intracapsular #
  ○ Inevitable interruption of intramedullary vessels, possible disruption to cervical arteries
  ○ Moderate risk of AVN
  ○ Usually pinned in the hope that AVN will not develop (~30% risk)
- Intertrochanteric or subtrochanteric extracapsular #
  ○ Little interruption to blood supply of femoral head
  ○ Low risk of AVN
  ○ Usually stabilised and reduced using dynamic hip screw

NOTES

Action / Examine for	ΔΔ / Potential findings / Extra information
Introduction	
• Wash hands	
• Introduce yourself, explain examination & gain consent	
• Expose & position pt (top off, standing)	
• " Do you have any pain in your back? Do you have any trouble walking?"	
Gait	
• Ask pt to walk across room, turn & walk back	[⇨ for gait abnormalities]
○ Note ease / steadiness of gait	
○ Abnormal posture	
○ Abnormal stride length / height	
Look	
• From front, sides and back	
○ Abnormal posture	
○ Muscle wasting	Chronic back pain, RA
○ Kyphosis	Ank spond, osteoporotic #, RA
○ Lordosis	Loss of lumbar lordosis in ank spond
○ Scoliosis	Idiopathic, neurofibromatosis
Feel	
• Spinous processes (entire length of spine, cervical to lumbar)	Bony tenderness / abnormality
• Sacroiliac joints	Sacroiliitis (e.g. ank spond)
• Paraspinal muscles	Tenderness, spasm
Move	
• Active movements only	Passive movements are sometimes performed on the cervical spine, but are not included in this sequence
• Cervical spine	
○ Lateral flexion – " Try to touch your ear to your shoulder"	
○ Flexion – " Put your chin down onto your chest"	
○ Extension – " Put your head back as far as possible"	
○ Rotation – " Look over your shoulder"	
• Lumbar spine	
○ Flexion – " Try to touch your toes"	
○ Extension – " Lean back as far as possible"	
○ Lateral flexion – " Lean to side, slide your hand down your leg"	
• Thoracic spine	
○ Pt sitting on side of bed (stabilises pelvis)	
○ Rotation – " Twist your shoulders round"	

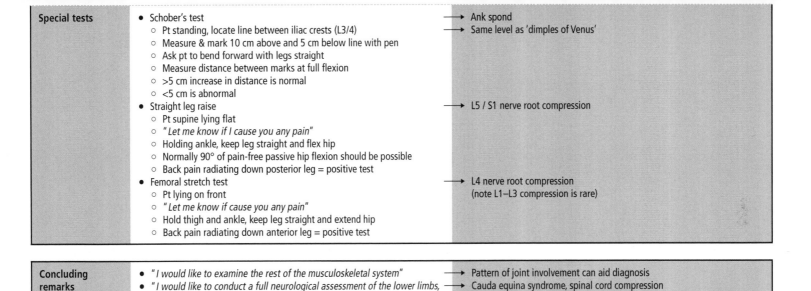

Special tests	• Schober's test	→ Ank spond
	○ Pt standing, locate line between iliac crests (L3/4)	→ Same level as 'dimples of Venus'
	○ Measure & mark 10 cm above and 5 cm below line with pen	
	○ Ask pt to bend forward with legs straight	
	○ Measure distance between marks at full flexion	
	○ >5 cm increase in distance is normal	
	○ <5 cm is abnormal	
	• Straight leg raise	→ L5 / S1 nerve root compression
	○ Pt supine lying flat	
	○ "Let me know if I cause you any pain"	
	○ Holding ankle, keep leg straight and flex hip	
	○ Normally 90° of pain-free passive hip flexion should be possible	
	○ Back pain radiating down posterior leg = positive test	
	• Femoral stretch test	→ L4 nerve root compression
	○ Pt lying on front	(note L1–L3 compression is rare)
	○ "Let me know if cause you any pain"	
	○ Hold thigh and ankle, keep leg straight and extend hip	
	○ Back pain radiating down anterior leg = positive test	

Concluding remarks	• "I would like to examine the rest of the musculoskeletal system"	→ Pattern of joint involvement can aid diagnosis
	• "I would like to conduct a full neurological assessment of the lower limbs, and perform a PR exam if indicated"	→ Cauda equina syndrome, spinal cord compression
	• Investigations: X-rays, MRI spine	

Ankylosing spondylitis

- Aetiology
  - Primary
  - Associated with psoriasis / IBD
- 5 males : 1 female (♂ usually severe disease)
- Presents in 20s
- Strong association with HLA-B27
- X-ray findings
  - Sacroiliitis
  - Bamboo spine
    - squaring of vertebrae
    - disc ossification
    - spinal fusion (syndesmophytes)
- Associated features
  - Uveitis
  - Peripheral enthesitis in 33% (especially Achilles tendonitis)
- Management
  - Simple analgesia
  - NSAIDs
  - Anti-TNFα therapy where NSAIDs fail

Neurogenic claudication

- Due to spinal stenosis (lumbosacral OA with narrowing of bony foramina & nerve root impingement)
- Calf / buttock / thigh discomfort when walking
- Classically relieved by bending forwards at waist (spinal flexion opens up bony foramina)
- This feature is useful in differentiating from intermittent (vascular) claudication

ΔΔ Lumbar back pain

- Mechanical
  - Muscular
  - Disc prolapse
  - OA
  - # (e.g. osteoporotic wedge #)
  - Spondylolisthesis (vertebral 'slipping')
  - Spinal stenosis
- Inflammatory
  - Ankylosing spondylitis
- Other serious pathology
  - Bone metastases
  - Myeloma
  - TB
  - Osteomyelitis

NOTES

Gait abnormalities

	Features	Causes
Antalgic	• Less time spent on painful limb (a limp)	• Pathology of hip / knee / ankle

Trendelenberg	• Waddling gait	• Hip ABductor weakness
		  ○ Nerve lesion
		  ○ Root lesion
		  ○ Muscular dystrophy
		  ○ Myopathy
		  ○ Polio
		• # NOF
		• CDH
		• SUFE

Parkinsonian
[p44]
	• Hesitation
	• Shuffling
	• Loss of arm swing
	• Hurried steps – 'marche à petit pas'
	• Festination (speeding up inadvertently)
	• Retropulsion (falling backwards as feet rush ahead)
		• Parkinsonism
		  ○ Parkinson's disease
		  ○ Drug-induced
		  ○ Parkinson-plus syndrome
		• Atherosclerotic pseudoparkinsonism

Sensory ataxic	• Broad-based
	• Looking at feet
		• Sensory peripheral neuropathy
		• Dorsal column loss
		  ○ MS
		  ○ SCDC
		  ○ Tabes dorsalis

Cerebellar [p48]	• Broad-based • High-stepping • Looking carefully ahead	• Cerebellar lesion (usually vermis)

Hemiplegic	• Foot plantarflexed and knee extended
	• Leg must be abducted and swung in a lateral arc
	• Arm may also be held in UMN posture
		• UMN lesion
		  ○ Stroke
		  ○ Tumour
		  ○ MS

Foot-drop	• High-stepping to allow toes to clear ground	• Common peroneal nerve palsy • Sciatic nerve palsy • L4 / L5 root lesion • MND • Peripheral motor neuropathy (e.g. alcoholic)

	Action / Examine for	ΔΔ / Potential findings / Extra information

Introduction	• Wash hands
	• Introduce yourself, explain examination & gain consent
	• Expose pt (fully from waist down)
	• Position: Dependent on scenario
	  ○ If pt already supine & swelling obvious, examine supine
	  ○ If pt already supine & swelling not obvious, examine standing
	  ○ If pt already standing, examine standing
	• *"Can you show me where you have you noticed the abnormality?"*
	• *"Is the lump painful"*
		→ Ensure privacy
		
		→ Herniae become more apparent on standing due to increased intra-abdominal pressure

Inspection	• Look for swellings on *both* sides • Scars (look carefully in groin creases) • *"Give me a loud cough"* – look for visible cough impulse	→ Previous surgical repair

Palpation	• Get down on one knee, keep checking pt's face
	• *"Let me know if you feel any discomfort"*
	• Start with quick feel of 'normal' side (if there is one)
	  ○ Palpable swelling
	  ○ Cough impulse
	• Move onto affected side
	  ○ Size of swelling
	  ○ Tension / heat / tenderness
	  ○ Try to locate lower extent of swelling
	  ○ Cough impulse
	• Locate pubic tubercle
	  ○ Hernia above tubercle = inguinal
	  ○ Hernia below tubercle = femoral
	• Palpate scrotum if ♂
	  ○ Extension of groin swelling
	  ○ Try to 'get above' any scrotal swelling
		→ May be a smaller, un-noticed hernia
		
		→ Strangulation
		→ If impossible may extend into scrotum
		→ If absent:
		  ○ Incarcerated hernia
		  ○ Alternative diagnosis
		    (lymph node, sebaceous cyst, lipoma, saphena varix)
		→ Usually indirect inguinal hernia
		→ If possible, swelling is not a hernia

Reduction	• Establish whether reducible
	  ○ Ask pt to reduce – *"Can you push the lump back inside?"*
	  ○ If unable, gently try to reduce yourself (with permission)
	  ○ If still unable and pt standing, try supine
	• Establish relationship to deep inguinal ring (if reducible)
	  ○ Reduce hernia
	  ○ Locate deep ring (half way between ASIS & pubic tubercle)
	  ○ Occlude deep ring with 2 fingers (and hernia still reduced)
	  ○ Ask pt to cough
	  ○ Does hernia reappear on coughing despite pressure on deep ring?
		→ Irreducible = incarcerated [⇨]
		
		→ The midpoint of the inguinal ligament
		
		→ Reappears = direct. Held by pressure = indirect

Auscultation	• Auscultate over lump for bowel sounds	→ Hernia contents: bowel or omentum

Concluding remarks	• If not done: "*I would like to examine the contralateral groin*" • If examined supine: "*I would like to examine the groins with the pt standing to check for a small hernia on the contralateral side*" • "*I would like to perform a full abdominal exam, in particular looking for a cause of raised intra-abdominal pressure*" → Hepatomegaly, splenomegaly, APKD, bladder distension, ascites, etc. → Exclude a cystic scrotal swelling • Transillumination of any scrotal mass

Definition of a hernia: The protrusion of whole or part of a viscus through an opening in the wall of its containing cavity into a place where it is not normally found.

Features of groin hernias

	Indirect inguinal	Direct inguinal	Femoral
Route of herniation (*Fig. 7*)	Through internal inguinal ring, down inguinal canal and out of external ring	Through weak point in posterior wall of inguinal canal (Hesselbach's triangle*)	Through femoral canal underneath inguinal ligament
Relationship to pubic tubercle	Superior	Superior	Inferior
Extension into scrotum	Common	Rare	Impossible
Size	Can be very large	Moderate	Normally 3–5 cm
Reducible	Usually	Almost always	Rare (usually incarcerated with absent cough impulse)
Held by pressure on deep ring	✓	✗	✗
Complications	Low risk of incarceration and complication	Moderate risk of incarceration and complication	Usually incarcerated with high risk of strangulation
Management	Usually repaired as it is impossible to be 100% sure hernia is indirect on basis of clinical examination alone	Surgical repair	Urgent surgical repair

* Borders of Hesselbach's triangle
- Inferior epigastric artery
- Inguinal ligament
- Linea semilunaris (lateral border of rectus muscle)

Types of surgical hernia repair
- Open mesh repair (Lichtenstein)
- Open suture repair (Babinski / Shouldice)
- Laparoscopic
  - TEP (total extraperitoneal procedure)
  - TAP (trans-abdominal procedure)

Risk factors for developing a hernia
- Family history
- Weakness of abdominal musculature
  - Increasing age (especially direct)
  - Surgery (incisional hernia)
- Increased intra-abdominal pressure
  - Obesity
  - Pregnancy
  - Other organomegaly
  - COPD / chronic cough
  - Prostatism
  - Constipation
  - Heavy lifting

NOTES

Complications of a hernia:

Incarceration (irreducible) <
1. Obstruction (clinically: colic, constipation, vomiting, distension)

2. Strangulation → ischaemia → necrosis → peritonitis

Richter's hernia
- Only part of the bowel wall herniates, allowing strangulation without obstruction
- More common in femoral hernia (narrower orifice)

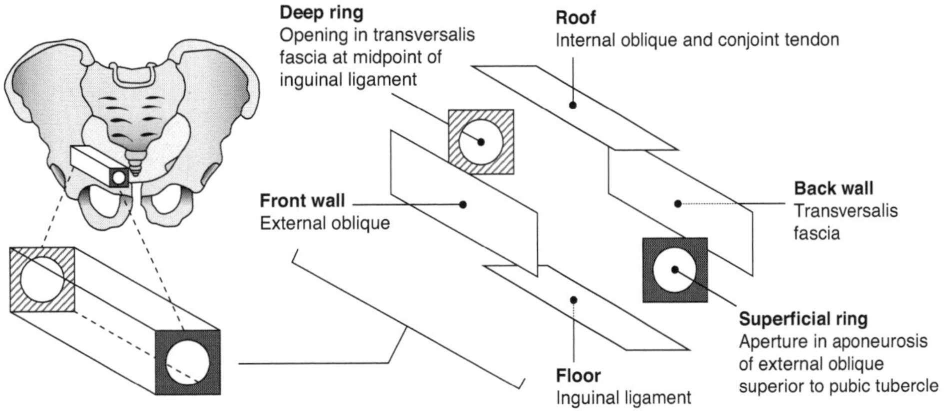

Deep ring
Opening in transversalis fascia at midpoint of inguinal ligament

Roof
Internal oblique and conjoint tendon

Front wall
External oblique

Back wall
Transversalis fascia

Superficial ring
Aperture in aponeurosis of external oblique superior to pubic tubercle

Floor
Inguinal ligament

Fig. 7. Anatomy of the inguinal canal

	Action / Examine for	ΔΔ / Potential findings / Extra information
Introduction	• Wash hands • Introduce yourself, explain examination & gain consent • Expose pt (entire neck)	→ Unbutton / remove top to see base of neck
End of bed	• Thin, fidgety, tremulous, sweaty, flushed, restless • Fat, warmly dressed, hair loss, dry skin, deep voice	→ Hyperthyroid → Hypothyroid

Thyroid / Neck lump		

Inspection	• *"Where is the area of concern?"*
	• Look from front & sides
	• Define location: midline, anterior / posterior triangle
	• Swallowing
	  ○ Ask pt to take sip of water and hold it in mouth
	  ○ Instruct to swallow as you look from front
	  ○ Repeat looking from side
	• Stick out tongue
		→ Narrows the ΔΔ [⇨]
		→ Thyroid moves upwards
		
		→ Thyroglossal cyst moves upwards

Palpation of neck lump	• *"Have you any pain in your neck?"*
	• Stand behind pt, use both hands to examine
	  ○ Start in centre of lump, move out to edges
	  ○ Size / shape / symmetry
	  ○ Surface
	  ○ Consistency
	  ○ Edge
	  ○ Fluctuance
	  ○ Pulsation
	• Specific to thyroid swelling
	  ○ Diffuse enlargement or single nodule?
	  ○ If diffuse, is it smooth or multinodular?
	  ○ Lower extent – can you get below thyroid?
	• Palpate from behind whilst pt swallows water
	• Attempt to transilluminate lump
		→ Goitre [⇨]
		  ○ Graves': soft, smooth, symmetrical
		  ○ MNG: firm, usually nodular, often asymmetrical (dominant nodule)
		
		→ Well defined, indistinct, irregular
		→ Lipoma
		→ Carotid body tumour
		
		→ If impossible goitre may extend retrosternally
		→ Thyroid moves on swallowing
		→ Neck cyst: thyroglossal, branchial, cystic hygroma

Palpation of nodes	• Always perform this • Palpate systematically standing behind pt [p111]	
Percussion	• Percuss sternum from xiphisternum up to suprasternal notch	→ Retrosternal goitre may cause dull percussion note
Auscultation	• Both sides of lump (ask pt to hold breath)	→ Bruit is virtually diagnostic of Graves'

Special tests	• Pemberton's test (if large goitre)
	  ○ Slowly raise both arms above head
	  ○ Watch for facial plethora
	  ○ *"Take a deep breath in"* – listen for stridor
		→ Thoracic inlet obstruction due to a large retrosternal goitre
		→ Obstructed venous return from head
		→ Tracheal compression

Thyroid status (assess in any pt with goitre or thyroid symptoms)		Hyperthyroid	Hypothyroid
Hands & wrist	• Acropachy (clubbing)	→ Graves' [p112 for ΔΔ]	
	• **P**alms	→ Hot, sweaty	→ Cold, dry
	• **P**almar erythema	→ Yes	
	• **P**aper (put on top of hands to detect fine tremor)	→ Yes	
	• **P**ulse	→ Tachycardia ± AF	→ Bradycardia
Face	• Facial appearance	→ Flushed	→ 'Peaches & cream'
	• Hair & eyebrows		→ Thin, brittle
	• Eyes	→ [⇨]	
	○ Exophthalmos	→ Graves'	
	○ Eyelids	→ Lid retraction	→ May be puffy
	• Eye movements		
	○ "Follow my finger; tell me if you see double"		
	○ Move in 'H' pattern		
	○ Look for obvious ophthalmoplegia (esp. upgaze)	→ Graves'	
	• Lid lag	→ Yes	
	○ Stand to side of pt		
	○ "Follow my finger, keep your head still"		
	○ Move finger upwards so you see lids retract		
	○ Quickly move finger downwards – look for delay in lids descending		
Limbs	• Knee & biceps reflexes	→ Brisk	→ Slow-relaxing
	• Carpal tunnel syndrome		→ Yes [p40]
	○ Median nerve power / sensation		
	○ Tinel / Phalen tests		
	• Proximal myopathy	→ Yes	
	○ Shoulder ABduction		
	○ Stand up from chair with arms crossed (hip girdle strength)		
	• Oedema		
	○ Pre-tibial myxoedema	→ Grave's	
	○ Generalised non-pitting peripheral oedema		→ Yes

Concluding remarks	• If not done: "I would like to assess thyroid status"
	• Investigations: TFTs, USS, FNA

ΔΔ Neck lump
- Midline
  - Goitre
  - Thyroglossal cyst
- Anterior triangle
  - Branchial cyst – under the top of SCM
  - Carotid body tumour
  - Lymph node [p111]
- Posterior triangle
  - Cystic hygroma (above clavicle)
  - Lymph node
- Anywhere
  - Sebaceous cyst
  - Lipoma [p102]

ΔΔ Goitre
- Multinodular goitre
- Graves' disease
- Solitary nodule (adenoma / carcinoma)
- Hashimoto's thyroiditis
- Subacute thyroiditis

ΔΔ Hypothyroidism
- Autoimmune
  - Primary atrophic thyroiditis (no goitre)
  - Hashimoto's initially
- Acquired
  - Iodine deficiency (no. 1 cause worldwide)
  - Subacute thyroiditis
  - Iatrogenic
    - surgery
    - radioiodine
    - carbimazole
    - lithium
    - amiodarone
- Secondary
  - Panhypopituitarism (*very rare*)

Multinodular goitre (MNG)
- Most common large goitre
- Rarely can be smooth rather than multinodular to feel
- Pt usually euthyroid = non-toxic MNG
- Hyperthyroid = toxic MNG
- Indications for surgery in non-toxic MNG
  - Cosmetic reasons
  - Local compression effect

Graves' disease
- Classic features
  - Goitre
  - Thyrotoxicosis
  - Eye disease (50%)
    - exophthalmos
    - ophthalmoplegia ⎫ Unique to
  - Pretibial myxoedema ⎬ Graves'
  - Thyroid acropachy ⎭
- Factors differentiating from toxic MNG
  - Smooth goitre (MNG rarely smooth)
  - Graves'-unique features as above
  - TSH-receptor antibodies
- Indications for surgery
  - Cosmetic reasons
  - Local compression effect
  - Failed medical Rx
  - Intolerant of medication

A note on thyroid eye signs
- Any cause of hyperthyroidism
  - Lid retraction
  - Lid lag
- Specific to Graves' disease
  - Exophthalmos
  - Ophthalmoplegia

NOTES

ΔΔ Hyperthyroidism
- Graves'
- Toxic MNG } 90%
- Toxic nodule (usually adenoma)
- Thyroiditis in the initial phase
  - Hashimoto's
  - Post-partum
  - Subacute
- Secondary (*rare*)
  - TSHoma
  - Hydatidiform mole
  - Choriocarcinoma

ΔΔ Parotid swelling
- Bilateral
  - Viral / bacterial parotitis
  - TB
  - Alcohol
  - Pleomorphic adenoma
  - Sjögren's
  - Sarcoidosis
- Unilateral
  - Duct blockage
  - Unilateral pleomorphic adenoma

Hyperthyroidism Rx
- Medical
  - Symptomatic control: β-blockers
  - Anti-thyroid therapy: carbimazole
- Radioiodine
- Surgical (cosmetic, compression, malignancy)
  - Total thyroidectomy
  - Subtotal thyroidectomy

Contraindications to radioiodine
- Pregnancy / breast feeding
- Young children at home
- Incontinent (eliminated in urine)

Complications of thyroidectomy
- Early
  - Anaesthetic / haemorrhage / infection
  - Damage to surrounding structures
    - recurrent laryngeal nerve
    - trachea
    - oesophagus
    - neck musculature
  - Transient hypoparathyroidism
- Late
  - Hypoparathyroidism
  - Recurrent hyperthyroidism
  - Hypothyroidism

NOTES

	Action / Examine for	ΔΔ / Potential findings / Extra information
Introduction	• Wash hands • Introduce yourself, explain examination & gain consent • Expose & position pt (down to pants or shorts, supine at 45°) • *"Are you sore anywhere in your legs or feet?"*	

Inspection	• Colour
	  ○ Pallor
	  ○ Mottling
	  ○ Redness with dependency
	  ○ Black
	• Peripheral oedema
	• Trophic changes
	  ○ Pale skin
	  ○ Hair loss
	  ○ Onychogryphosis
	  ○ Fungal infections (skin / nails)
	• Guttering of superficial veins
	• Ulcers
	  ○ Site
	  ○ Edge
	  ○ Exudate
	• Scars
	• Quickly look for abdominal scars
		→ Ischaemia (especially acute)
		→ Acute ischaemia (unlikely in OSCE!)
		→ Chronic ischaemia [⇨]
		→ Tissue necrosis / gangrene
		→ Venous disease [p113]
		→ Chronic arterial disease
		
		→ Thickened, distorted nail
		
		→ Chronic arterial disease
		→ [⇨ for arterial vs. venous]
		
		→ Fem-pop bypass, fem-distal bypass
		→ Aorto-bifemoral graft

Palpation	• Temperature
	  ○ Use back of hand
	  ○ Compare sides
	  ○ Use one of your hands only (i.e. *not* both hands at once)
	• Capillary refill time
	  ○ Increased
	  ○ Reduced
		→ Cold implies arterial insufficiency
		
		→ Normally 1–2 sec
		→ PVD / ischaemia
		→ Dependent blood pooling [⇨]

Pulses	• Always move from proximal to distal
	• Assess rate, rhythm, character & symmetry
	• Move from side to side
	• Femoral
	  ○ Half-way between ASIS & pubic symphysis
	  ○ Below inguinal ligament
	  ○ Demonstrate use of surface anatomy
	  ○ Auscultate for femoral bruits
	• Popliteal
	  ○ Flex knee to 30°, ensure pt relaxed
	  ○ Grasp knee with both hands, thumbs in front, feel with fingers
	• Posterior tibial
	  ○ Behind medial malleolus
	• Dorsalis pedis
	  ○ Between bases of 1st & 2nd metatarsals
		→ Mid-inguinal point
		
		→ Femoral artery disease
		→ Often hard to feel – don't worry if you can't (and don't pretend you can!)

Special tests	• Buerger's test
	  ○ Lie pt flat
	  ○ Normal side first
	  ○ Slowly perform straight leg raise
	  ○ Look for 'guttering' of superficial veins
	  ○ Note point at which leg goes pale – angle between leg and the horizontal at this point is 'Buerger's angle'
	• Quick version (if short of time)
	  ○ Lift leg straight up to ~70° hip flexion
	  ○ Assess capillary refill time
		→ Shallower angle = more severe PVD
		
		→ Increased in PVD

Concluding remarks	• Measure BP
	• Measure ankle-brachial pressure index
	• Assess for risk factors for peripheral arterial disease
	  ○ Tar staining on hands
	  ○ Stigmata of hypercholesterolaemia
	• Further investigations: Doppler USS, MRA
		→ [⇨]

Beware the pt with one red foot and one pale foot (often with *rapid* CRT in the red foot)
- Easy to think the white foot is the ischaemic one
- In fact the whiter foot may be normal, with the red foot occurring due to dependent pooling of venous blood in a chronically ischaemic limb (the pt may have been sitting up in a chair prior to your arrival)
- Before commenting, feel the temperature of the feet and see what happens to the red foot when it is elevated from the bed – if ischaemic it will rapidly exsanguinate and become very pale

Causes of 'claudication' in presence of normal peripheral pulses:
1. Neurogenic claudication (spinal stenosis)
2. Anaemia
3. β-blockers

Critically ischaemic limb (6 Ps)
- **P**ain
- **P**allor
- **P**ulseless
- **P**erishingly cold
- **P**araesthesia
- **P**aralysis (best indicator of danger to limb)

ABPI measurements
- >1   Normal
- 0.5–1   Intermittent claudication
- 0.3–0.5   Rest pain / critical limb ischaemia
- <0.3   Gangrene + ulceration

Arterial supply to the lower limbs

Common iliac → Internal iliac
Common iliac → External iliac → (Inguinal ligament) → Common femoral → Superficial femoral → Popliteal → (Popliteal trifurcation) → Anterior tibial → Dorsalis pedis
Common femoral → Deep femoral (profunda femoris)
Popliteal → Posterior tibial
Popliteal → Peroneal

Leriche's syndrome: Bilateral buttock pain and erectile impotence due to common iliac disease

NOTES

	Venous ulcer [p94]	Arterial ulcer
History	• Varicose veins • DVTs	• Intermittent claudication • Rest pain
Classic sites	• Medial gaiter region of lower leg	• Feet / toes • Ankle (lateral maleolus)
Edges	• Sloped	• Punched-out
Exudate	• Lots	• Usually little
Pain	• Not severe unless associated with excessive oedema or infection	• Painful
Oedema	• Usually associated with limb oedema	• Oedema uncommon
Associated features	• Venous eczema • Haemosiderosis • Lipodermatosclerosis • Atrophie blanche	• Trophic changes • Gangrene

Management	• Graduated compression dressing
	• Antibiotics for infection
		• Conservative
		• Endovascular revascularisation (angioplasty)
		• Surgical revascularisation
		  ○ Depends on sites of disease
		  ○ Fem-pop bypass
		  ○ Fem-distal bypass
		  ○ Axillo-femoral bypass
		  ○ Aorto-bifemoral graft

Diabetic foot features
- Peripheral neuropathy
  ○ Loss of ankle jerk and vibration sense
  ○ Accidental injury / tissue damage*
  ○ Charcot joints (neuropathic arthropathy)
- Large vessel arterial disease*
- Small vessel arterial disease*

- Autonomic neuropathy
  ○ Reduced sweating
  ○ Dry, cracked skin*
  ○ Infection*

*contribute to ulcer formation

NOTES

_____

_____

_____

_____

_____

Action / Examine for	ΔΔ / Potential findings / Extra information
Introduction	
• Wash hands	
• Introduce yourself, explain examination & gain consent	
• Expose & position pt (down to pants or shorts, standing)	
• *"Are you sore anywhere in your legs or feet?"*	
Inspection	
• Varicose veins	
○ Posterior lower leg	→ Short saphenous system
○ Medial lower leg & thigh	→ Long saphenous system
• Saphena varix	→ Dilated SFJ (2° incompetence)
○ Blue-ish lump in groin apparent when standing	→ Usually disappears when supine
• Signs of progressive chronic venous insufficiency	[p113 for ΔΔ]
○ Oedema	
○ Venous eczema	
○ Haemosiderosis	→ Very common – extravasation of haemosiderin (a blood breakdown product) due to venous hypertension
■ brown speckled discoloration	
■ 'cayenne pepper petechiae'	
■ especially medial gaiter area	
○ Lipodermatosclerosis	→ Disproportionately narrow ankles
■ scarring of subcutaneous fat	
■ skin tight and indurated	
■ may cause 'inverted champagne bottle' legs	
○ Atrophie blanche	
■ white scar-like areas	→ [p91 for features]
○ Ulceration	
■ especially medial gaiter area	
(progression ↑)	
Palpation	
• Skin texture for lipodermatosclerosis	
○ Hard	
○ 'Woody'	
• Calf tenderness	→ DVT
• Varicose veins	
○ Tenderness	→ Superficial phlebitis
○ Temperature (warmth)	→ Superficial phlebitis
• Saphenofemoral incompetence	
○ Locate pubic tubercle	
○ Approximate position of SFJ is 2 cm inferior & lateral	
○ May be marked by presence of saphena varix	
○ With fingers in this position (or on varix) ask pt to cough	
○ Feel for cough impulse – if present +ve test	

Special tests	• Trendelenburg (tourniquet) test	→ Identifies level of venous incompetence
	○ Have pt lie flat	
	○ Perform straight leg raise & put leg on your shoulder	
	○ Expedite emptying of veins by stroking them towards groin	
	○ Once empty, apply tourniquet tightly in upper thigh	
	○ Have pt stand up	
	○ Look for varicosities filling for 10–15 sec then release tourniquet	
	○ 2 common outcomes	
	▪ no filling on standing & rapid filling on release of tourniquet	→ Isolated sapheno-femoral junction incompetence
	▪ slow filling on standing & rapid filling on release of tourniquet	→ Mixed sapheno-femoral junction and perforating vein incompetence

Concluding remarks	• Examine the lower limb arterial system	→ Ulcers may be multifactorial
	• Perform Perthes test	→ Distinguish antegrade & retrograde flow in superficial varices
	• Further investigations: Doppler USS to identify sites of incompetence	

How to present your findings

In the common case of a patient with obvious varicose veins
- There are varicose veins in the distribution of the [long / short / both] saphenous systems
- There [is / is no] saphena varix
- Trendelenburg test suggests [sapheno-femoral / mixed sapheno-femoral and perforator] incompetence
- There [are / are no] associated features of chronic venous insufficiency
- There [is / is no] evidence of superficial thrombophlebitis

Example: The pt has varicose veins of both legs in the distribution of the long saphenous systems. There are saphena varices bilaterally with positive cough impulses. The Trendelenburg test indicates isolated sapheno-femoral incompetence. There are associated features of chronic venous insufficiency, namely oedema, haemosiderosis and lipodermatosclerosis. There is no evidence of superficial thrombophlebitis.

Varicose veins

- Occur as a result of valvular incompetence
  - Structural predisposition (familial tendency)
  - Factors that ↑ venous pressure: prolonged standing, obesity, pregnancy
- Sites of incompetence
  - Sapheno-femoral junction (SFJ) – typically causes long saphenous vein (LSV) varices
  - Sapheno-popliteal junction (SPJ) – typically causes short saphenous vein (SSV) varices
  - Perforating veins linking deep veins and saphenous systems
- Often associated with signs of chronic venous insufficiency [see over]

Management of varicose veins

- Conservative
  - Elastic support hose
  - Weight loss
  - Regular exercise
  - Avoid prolonged standing
- Injection sclerotherapy
  - Suitable for small varices below knee due to incompetence of local perforators
  - Not satisfactory for varices associated with SFJ incompetence (recurrence inevitable)
- Surgery
  - SFJ incompetence & LSV varices
    - SFJ ligated (a so-called 'high tie')
    - LSV usually stripped from knee to groin (reduced chance of recurrence)
    - stab avulsions of remaining varices
  - SPJ incompetence & SSV varices
    - SPJ ligated (SSV not stripped due to risk of damaging sural nerve)
    - stab avulsions of remaining varices
- New techniques
  - Ultrasound-guided foam sclerotherapy
  - Radiofrequency or laser obliteration of LSV / SSV

NOTES

Causes of chronic venous insufficiency
1. Valvular incompetence of deep veins (90%)
   - Primary (aetiology same as for varicose veins)
   - Secondary (damaged by DVT)
2. Obstruction of deep veins by DVT (10%)

Chronic venous insufficiency 2° DVT = 'post-thrombotic syndrome'

Superficial thrombophlebitis
- Inflammation and thrombosis almost invariably occurring in varicose veins
- Redness and tenderness follow line of vein
- Thrombosis may spread to deep system and cause DVT
- Management
  - Analgesia
  - NSAIDs
  - Support stockings
  - Active exercise
- Underlying vein usually removed as recurrence is common
- Propagation towards deep veins is an indication for IV heparin

Breast Examination

	Action / Examine for	ΔΔ / Potential findings / Extra information
Introduction	• Wash hands • Introduce yourself, explain examination & gain consent • Offer chaperone • Expose & position pt (top and bra off, sitting on side of bed) • *"Have you noticed any breast lumps? Where is the area of concern?"*	

Inspection	• Obvious lump
	• Skin changes
	• Scars from previous surgery
	  ○ Breasts
	  ○ Axillae
	• Compare breasts
	  ○ Hands resting by side
	  ○ Hands pushing down on bed
	  ○ Hands pushing in on hips
	  ○ Slowly raise straight arms up above head
	• Nipples
	  ○ Inversion
	  ○ Discharge
	  ○ Paget's disease of the nipple
		→ Dimpling, peau d'orange
		
		→ Mastectomy, lumpectomy
		→ Axillary node clearance
		
		→ May reveal dimpling [⇨]
		→ May reveal dimpling [⇨]
		→ May reveal dimpling [⇨]
		
		→ Advanced malignant disease, normal variant
		→ Note colour, blood-staining
		→ Intraductal carcinoma

Palpation	• Position pt lying flat with hands behind head
	• *"Let me know if I cause you any discomfort"*
	• Assess each breast in turn – 'normal' one first
	  ○ Use pads of middle 3 fingers
	  ○ Move systematically (e.g. 'clock face')
	  ○ If lump found, assess as you would any other lump
	  ○ Axillary tail
	• Axillary lymph nodes
	• Lymph nodes of head & neck
		
		→ [p100]
		
		→ [p111]

Concluding remarks	• If not done: *"I would like to examine the other breast"*
	• If lump identified: *"I would go on to complete triple assessment of the breast lump"*
	  ○ Imaging (mammography / USS)
	  ○ Fine needle aspiration	

Examination of the Male Genitalia

	Action / Examine for	ΔΔ / Potential findings / Extra information
Introduction	• Wash hands • Introduce yourself, explain examination & gain consent • Offer chaperone • Expose & position pt (underwear removed, lying flat with 1 pillow) • *"Have you noticed any lumps in your testes? Have you had any pain in your testes? Could you point to the area of concern?"*	

Inspection	• Testes
	  ○ Enlargement / obvious mass
	  ○ Skin changes
	• Penis, groins & thighs
	  ○ Rash / infestation
	• Ask pt to retract foreskin & inspect glans / prepuce
	  ○ Rashes
	  ○ Discharge
		→ Tinea, pubic lice (a highly unlikely and extremely harsh OSCE case!)

Palpation	• Wear gloves
	• Examine each testis in turn – 'normal' one first
	• Palpate testis with both hands between thumb and index finger
	  ○ Swelling / irregularity
	  ○ Tenderness
	• Identify spermatic cord and epididymis
	• Palpate rest of scrotum
	• If swelling identified
	  ○ Attempt to get above it
	  ○ Assess groins for swelling
	  ○ Identify if attached / separate to testis
	  ○ Transilluminate with torch
	• Examine with pt standing
		→ Hard / soft / fluctuant / 'bag of worms' (varicocoele)
		
		→ If possible excludes inguinal hernia
		→ Hernia
		→ [⇨]
		→ Hydrocoele, epididymal cyst
		→ Varicocoele more obvious

Concluding remarks	• If malignancy suspected: *"I would like to perform a full systemic examination to look for evidence of metastatic disease"* • Investigations: USS, aspiration, bloods including HCG / αFP	→ [⇨]

Breast Examination

ΔΔ Breast lump
- Malignant (invasive ductal carcinoma most common)
- Benign
  - Fibroadenoma
  - Breast cyst (may be painful)
  - Abscess (painful, hot & swollen breast)

Triple assessment of a breast lump
1. Clinical examination
2. Imaging (USS / mammography)
3. Fine needle aspiration

Breast dimpling
- Does not necessarily imply invasion of cancer into underlying musculature
- Intra-mammary tumour can pull on a 'ligament of Astley Cooper', causing dimpling of the skin
- The action of raising the hands above the head tends to accentuate this

Breast cancer Rx
- Surgery
  - Lumpectomy
  - Wide local excision (if ≤4 cm tumour)
  - Partial mastectomy
  - Total mastectomy
    - axillary clearance if clinically node +ve
    - sentinel node biopsy if clinically node –ve → axillary clearance if biopsy +ve
  - Radical mastectomy (underlying musculature removed, axillary clearance)
- Chemotherapy
  - Greatest benefit in young, node +ve pts
- Radiotherapy
  - Sometimes used in WLE / partial mastectomy / node +ve disease
  - Not routinely used in total mastectomy
- Tamoxifen
  - Given to nearly all pts
  - Greatest benefit in oestrogen receptor & progesterone receptor +ve tumours
  - Avoid in pre-menopausal oestrogen receptor –ve pts (side-effects)

Examination of the Male Genitalia

ΔΔ Scrotal swelling:

	Tumour	Hydrocoele	Epididymal cyst	Varicocoele
Characteristics	Firm mass	Soft & smooth (may be large)	Soft & smooth	'Bag of worms'
Relationship to testis	Continuous	Continuous	Separate	Separate
Transillumination	–	✓✓	✓	–
Other information	Seminoma or teratoma	May be due to underlying tumour (aspirate & USS to exclude) Rarely congenital	Also known as spermatocoele	Examine pt standing (may disappear when supine) More common on left* ↑ incidence of infertility Rarely due to renal Ca*

Investigation of scrotal swelling
- USS
- Aspiration of fluid
- Tumour markers if malignancy suspected
  - αFP
  - βHCG

*Varicocoele more common on left side
- Right spermatic vein drains into IVC
  - Short, direct course
  - Lower incidence of valvular pathology
- Left spermatic vein drains into left renal vein
  - Long, tortuous course
  - Valves often absent or incompetent
  - Rarely, obstructed by renal Ca – new diagnosis of left variocoele requires an abdominal USS to exclude

Testicular tumours
- Rare
- Lymphatic spread to lungs and liver
- Rx orchidectomy + chemotherapy or radiotherapy
- Seminoma (60%) – Lance Armstrong
  - Age 30–40
  - Highly radiosensitive
  - 95% 5-year survival
- Teratoma (40%)
  - Age 20–30
  - Raised αFP in most
  - Raised β-HCG in many
  - Chemotherapy used
  - 75% 5-year survival – "terrible teratoma of the twenties"

NOTES

Examination of a Lump

	Action / Examine for	ΔΔ / Potential findings / Extra information
Introduction	• Wash hands • Introduce yourself, explain examination & gain consent • *"Where have you noticed the lump? Are there any more anywhere?"* • Expose relevant areas & position pt so comfortable	

Inspection	• Site
	• Relationship to surrounding anatomical structures
	• General idea of size and shape
	• Overlying skin
	  ○ Colour
	  ○ Punctum
	  ○ Discharge
		
		→ Better assessed by palpation
		
		→ Erythema
		→ Typical of sebaceous cyst
		→ Abscess

Palpation of lump	• *"Tell me if you feel any discomfort"*
	• Put your fingers on the centre of the lump
	  ○ Surface
	  ○ Consistency
	  ○ Heat
	  ○ Tenderness
	• Move to the borders
	  ○ Shape
	  ○ Size
	  ○ Edge
	• Assess fluctuance
	  ○ 'Bounce' lump between your two index fingers
	• Attachment to skin
	  ○ Try to slide skin over the lump
	• Attachment to other structures
	  ○ Ask pt to assume a position that contracts the underlying musculature – try to move lump
	  ○ If suspicious of a ganglion, ask pt to move joint that involves that particular tendon & feel if lump moves too
	• Feel for special characteristics
	  ○ Thrill
	  ○ Pulsation
	• Transilluminate with pen torch
		
		→ Smooth, irregular, craggy
		→ Hard, firm, rubbery, soft
		→ Inflammation
		→ Inflammation
		
		→ Circular, oblong, 'pear-shaped', etc.
		→ Estimate in cm
		→ Well-defined, indistinct, irregular
		
		→ Lipomas are fluctuant
		
		→ Impossible if intradermal [⇨]
		
		→ Attachment to musculature is suspicious of malignancy
		→ Ganglion will move with tendon of origin
		
		→ AV fistula
		→ Aneurysm
		→ Cystic swelling

	Action / Examine for	ΔΔ / Potential findings / Extra information

Palpation of nodes	• Palpate regional lymph nodes, especially if suspicion of malignancy
	  ○ Head & neck [p111 for technique]
	  ○ Axillary
	  ○ Groin	

Auscultation	• If palpable thrill or pulsation	→ Bruit in AV fistula

Concluding remarks	• If not done: "*I would like to assess for regional lymphadenopathy*"
	• "*I would enquire about any changes which might raise suspicion of a malignant lump*"
	  ○ Increasing size
	  ○ Changing surface / consistency / edge
	  ○ Development of associated pain
	• Investigations: FNA, imaging
		→ May be due to local invasion

Examination of a Skin Lesion

	Action / Examine for	ΔΔ / Potential findings / Extra information
Introduction	• Wash hands • Introduce yourself, explain examination & gain consent • "*Have you noticed any abnormalities of your skin? Where?*" • Expose relevant areas & position pt so comfortable	
Inspection	• Site or distribution if multiple lesions • Size • Shape • Border • Colour • Discharge	→ Single lesion / rash → Regular, irregular, 'rolled' (BCC) → Erythema
Palpation	• Feel if elevated above surrounding skin • Tenderness • Heat	→ Macule (flat) / papule (elevated) → Inflammation → Inflammation

Concluding remarks	• "*I would like to examine the rest of the pt's skin as well as performing a full systemic examination.*" • Investigations: bloods, biopsy, serial photographs	

Examination of a Lump

Intradermal lumps (impossible to slide skin over)
- Sebaceous cyst
- Abscess
- Dermoid cyst
- Granuloma

Subcutaneous lumps (skin can slide over)
- Lipoma
- Ganglion
- Neurofibroma
- Lymph node [p110]

Signs of inflammation
- Calor (heat)
- Dolor (pain)
- Rubor (erythema)
- Tumor (swelling)
- Loss of function

NOTES

Common benign lumps

	Lipoma	Sebaceous cyst	Ganglion
Description	Benign fatty tumour	Epidermal proliferation within dermis	Degenerative cyst from synovum of joint / tendon
Common sites	Anywhere fat can expand (*not* scalp or palms)	Anywhere on body (most common on trunk, neck, face & scalp)	Dorsum of hand / wrist Dorsal foot
Depth	Subcutaneous	Intradermal	Subcutaneous
Other features	Smooth Imprecise margins Fluctuant	Central punctum	Moves with tendon May transilluminate
Complications	Symptoms 2° pressure effects Malignant change (*very rare*)	Infection common	Rare
Management	Conservative Excision for cosmetic reasons or local pressure effects	Incision & drainage if infected Occasionally antibiotics needed Non-infected cysts can be 'shelled out' under local anaesthesia	Conservative (50% disappear) Aspiration Excision 'Blow from Bible' (not advised!)

Examination of a Skin Lesion

Common skin lesions
- Melanocytic naevus (mole)
- Urticaria
- Eczema
- Ulcers [see below]
- Spider naevi
- Campbell de Morgan spots
- Striae (e.g. Cushing's syndrome)
- Skin tags
- Psoriasis
- Seborrhoeic keratosis
- Erythema nodosum [p15]
- Tumour
  - Melanoma
  - Squamous cell carcinoma
  - Basal cell carcinoma
- Neurofibromatosis (common in OSCEs!)
  - Neurofibromata
  - Café au lait spots

ΔΔ Erythema nodosum
Painful, purple, raised lesions on shins
- Idiopathic (up to 55% of cases)
- Sarcoidosis (30–40% of cases)
- Infection
  - *Streptococci*
  - TB
- IBD
- Drugs
  - OCP
  - Sulphonamides
- Malignancy
  - Lymphoma
  - Leukaemia
- Pregnancy

Neurofibromatosis
- Genetic disorder
- 2 variants (Type 1 & Type 2)
- Both types autosomal dominant
- Type 1 = von Recklinghausen's disease (this neurofibroma **CATCHES** on my clothes)
  - **C**afé au lait patches (>6 is diagnostic)
  - **A**xillary freckling
  - **T**umours of nervous system
  - **C**utaneous neurofibromata
  - **H**ypertension
  - **E**ye features (Lisch nodules)
  - **S**coliosis
- Type 2
  - Bilateral acoustic neuromas (key feature)
  - Other tumours of nervous system
  - Fewer cutaneous features

ΔΔ Ulcer by type of edge
- Sloping   Venous   ⎤
- Punched-out Arterial   ⎬ [p91]
- Undermined   TB, pressure necrosis
- Rolling   Basal cell carcinoma
- Everted   Squamous cell carcinoma

Warning signs of a melanoma (ABCDE)
- **A**symmetry
- **B**order irregularity
- **C**olour variation
- **D**iameter (>6 mm or increasing)
- **E**levation

Examination of a Stoma

	Action / Examine for	ΔΔ / Potential findings / Extra information
Introduction	• Wash hands • Introduce yourself, explain examination & obtain consent • Expose pt (xiphisternum to pubic symphysis) • Position pt (supine at 45°) • *"Do you have any pain in your tummy?"* • *"Have you had any problems with your stoma?"*	

Inspection	• Site
	   ○ Left side of abdomen
	   ○ Right side of abdomen
	• Number of lumens
	• Spout
	• Effluent – *feel* the bag
	   ○ Hard stool
	   ○ Soft stool
	   ○ Urine
	• Surrounding skin quality
	• Complications
		[⇨ for features of stoma types]
		
		→ Inflammation / excoriation
		→ [⇨]

Auscultation	• Bowel sounds – just below umbilicus	→ Obstruction is a possible complication
Concluding remarks	• Stoma output chart • *"I would like to complete a full gastrointestinal & genitourinal examination"*	→ High or low output → As appropriate

	Action / Examine for	ΔΔ / Potential findings / Extra information
Introduction	<ul><li>Wash hands</li><li>Introduce yourself, explain examination & obtain consent</li><li>Expose pt (xiphisternum to pubic symphysis)</li><li>Position pt (standing or supine depending on situation – p80)</li><li>*"Where have you noticed the abnormality? Is it painful?"*</li></ul>	
Inspection	<ul><li>Scars</li><li>*"Give me a loud cough"* – look for visible cough impulse</li><li>Ask pt to lift head off bed<ul><li>Accentuates hernia (especially incisional)</li><li>Rectus divarication</li></ul></li></ul>	→ Incisional hernia → Increases intra-abdominal pressure → Weakness of linea alba (common) [⇨]
Palpation	<ul><li>*"Let me know if you feel any discomfort"*<ul><li>Size of swelling</li><li>Tension / temperature / tenderness</li><li>Cough impulse</li></ul></li></ul>	 → Strangulation → Absent = incarcerated / not a hernia
Reduction	<ul><li>Establish whether reducible<ul><li>Ask pt to reduce – *"Can you push that lump back inside for me?"*</li><li>If unable, gently try to reduce yourself (with permission)</li><li>If still unable and pt standing, try supine</li></ul></li></ul>	 → Irreducible = incarcerated
Auscultation	<ul><li>Auscultate over lump for bowel sounds</li></ul>	→ Hernia contents: bowel or omentum

Concluding remarks	<ul><li>If examined supine: *"I would now like to examine the patient standing"*</li><li>*"I would like to perform a full abdominal exam, in particular looking for a cause of raised intra-abdominal pressure"*</li><li>Investigations: abdominal wall USS, CT abdomen</li></ul>	→ Hepatomegaly, splenomegaly, APKD, bladder distension, ascites, etc.

Examination of a Stoma

How to present your findings (stoma)

To present your findings, run through the following order
1. Site
2. Number of lumens
3. Spout / flush with skin
4. Nature of effluent
5. State of surrounding skin
6. Evidence of complication
7. Likely type of stoma
8. Possible procedure / underlying pathology

Example: The pt has a stoma in the left iliac fossa with a single lumen, which is flush with the skin and producing hard faeces. The surrounding skin is intact and shows no evidence of inflammation. There is no evidence of any other stoma complication. This is most likely an end-colostomy which usually follows abdomino-perineal resection or Hartmann's procedure. The indication may have been a rectal malignancy. I would like to go on and perform a full gastrointestinal examination, and inquire as to whether the pt still has an anus [see below].

Features of different stoma types

	Site	Lumens	Spout	Effluent	Possible procedure
End colostomy*	Usually left	1	✗	Hard stool	→ Abdomino-perineal (AP) resection → Hartmann's procedure with rectum oversewn
End ileostomy	Usually right	1	✓	Soft or liquid stool	→ Panproctocolectomy (e.g. UC, FAP) → Emergency subtotal colectomy

Loop ileostomy (usually temporary)	Usually right	2 (joined)	✓	Soft or liquid stool	→ To defunction
					   ○ Obstruction (e.g. malignancy)
					   ○ Anus (e.g. Crohn's)
					   ○ Newly formed anastamosis

Loop colostomy (now rarely performed)	Upper abdomen	2 (joined)	✗	Hard stool	→ As above
End colostomy & mucous fistula	Usually left	2 (separate)	✗	Hard stool	→ Hartmann's procedure with rectum brought to skin
Urostomy	Either side	1	✓	Urine	→ Cystectomy (e.g. malignancy)

*If pt has an end-colostomy
- Ask: *"Do you mind telling me if you still have a back passage following your operation?"*
- No = AP resection for low rectal tumour
- Yes = Hartmann's procedure for higher tumour

Ideal site for a stoma
- Healthy skin
- Away from umbilicus & belt line
- Avoid
  - Bony prominences
  - Scars
  - Skin creases

Stoma complications
- Haemorrhage
- Necrosis
- Prolapse
- Retraction
- Obstruction
- Peristomal skin inflammation
- Parastomal hernia
- High output

Examination of a Ventral Hernia

Definition of a hernia: The protrusion of whole or part of a viscus through an opening in the wall of its containing cavity into a place where it is not normally found.

	Features	Surgical indications
Para-umbilical (acquired)	• Through linea alba, usually above umbilicus (rarely below) • Often irreducible	Always repaired (high risk of incarceration)
True umblical (congenital)	• Through umbilicus • Usually resolve spontaneously in early life	Indicated if persists at age 3
Epigastric	• Through linea alba in epigastrium • More common in thin individuals • 20% multiple, 80% just off midline	Usually repaired (moderate risk of incarceration)
Spigelian	• Through linea semilunaris at outer border of rectus sheath	Always repaired (high risk)
Incisional	• Can occur anywhere but especially midline surgery • Usually enlarge progressively & become cosmetic problem	Incarceration Cosmetic issues
Rectus divarication	• Not actually a hernia • Weakness of linea alba leads to bulge in epigastrium • Sometimes associated with paraumbilical & epigastric hernias	Cosmetic issues

APPENDICES

Lymph node groups

Pre-auricular
Posterior auricular
Occipital
Posterior cervical chain
Submental
Submandibular
Anterior cervical chain
Sternocleidomastoid
Supraclavicular

Virchow's node: enlarged left supraclavicular node due to metastasis of visceral (clasically gastric) malignancy

ΔΔ Lymphadenopathy
1. Localised
   - Acute local infection (e.g. tonsillitis)
   - Neoplastic
     - Local malignancy
     - Solitary distant metastasis
2. Generalised
   - Acute generalised infection
     - EBV
     - HIV seroconversion
   - Chronic infection
     - TB 'cold abscesses'
     - Syphilis
     - HIV
   - Neoplastic
     - Multiple distant metastases
     - Haematological
       - lymphoma
       - CLL
   - Systemic disease
     - Sarcoidosis
     - RA

Typical characteristics of lymphadenopathy
- Tender & fluctuant: Acute infection
- Non-tender & rubbery: Lymphoma / CLL
- Non-tender & hard: Metastatic

Examining the lymph nodes of the head and neck

Examination of the lymph nodes of the head and neck is a key component of several examinations. To begin, stand behind the pt and place both hands under their chin (over the submental nodes). Using the pads of your index, middle and ring fingers feel carefully in the sequence shown below. Examine both sides simultaneously. If you detect lymphadenopathy, assess the enlarged lymph node as you would any other lump [p100].

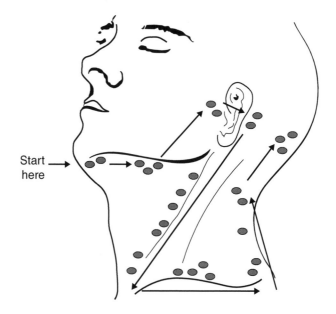

Start here →

Recommended sequence of lymph node palpation

1. Submental
2. Submandibular
3. Pre-auricular
4. Posterior auricular
5. Anterior cervical chain
6. Supraclavicular
7. Posterior cervical chain
8. Occipital

The following clinical signs come up time and time again due to their association with various diseases of multiple systems. Their causes are essential to know verbatim.

Features of finger clubbing
- Increased fluctuance of nailbed
- Loss of nailbed angle
- Increased longitudinal curvature of nail
- Drumsticking

ΔΔ Finger clubbing
Systems implicated: cardiovascular, respiratory, gastrointestinal, endocrine

- Cardiovascular disease
  - Cyanotic congenital heart disease
  - Infective endocarditis
  - Atrial myxoma

- Respiratory disease
  - Interstitial lung disease
  - Malignancy
    - bronchogenic carcinoma
    - mesothelioma
  - Suppurative lung disease
    - bronchiectasis (*pus in the tubes*)
    - abscess (*pus in a collection*)
    - empyema (*pus outside the lung*)
    - cystic fibrosis (*pus everywhere*)

- Gastrointestinal disease
  - IBD
  - Hepatic cirrhosis
  - GI lymphoma
  - Coeliac disease

- Other causes
  - Thyroid acropachy (Graves' disease)
  - Familial

ΔΔ Ankle swelling
Systems implicated: cardiovascular, respiratory, gastrointestinal, renal, endocrine, vascular

- Pitting oedema
  - Raised venous pressure
    - chronic venous insufficiency
    - right heart failure
    - volume overload (e.g. renal failure)
    - immobility
    - constrictive pericarditis
    - obesity (with associated Na$^+$ / H$_2$O retention)
    - pregnancy
  - Reduced oncotic pressure (hypoalbuminaemia)
    - nephrotic syndrome
    - cirrhosis / liver failure
    - severe malnutrition
    - protein-losing enteropathy (e.g. IBD)
    - exfoliative dermatitis
  - Drug-related
    - calcium channel blockers
    - long-term corticosteroids [p52]
    - NSAIDs

- Non-pitting oedema
  - Lymphoedema
    - primary (e.g. Milroy's disease)
    - malignancy
    - filariasis
    - radiotherapy
    - lymph node clearance
  - Hypothyroidism
  - Pre-tibial myxoedema (Graves' disease)

- Unilateral / localised swelling
  - Acute DVT
  - Post-thrombotic syndrome
  - Associated with cellulitis